THE

BEVERLY HILLS

RECIPES
TO
FOREVER

JUDY MAZEL

Health Communications, Inc.
Deerfield Beach, Florida

www.hci-online.com

Recipes to Forever and *The New Beverly Hills Diet* are not intended as a substitute for the medical advice of physicians. The reader should regularly consult a physician in matters relating to his or her health and especially with respect to any symptoms that may require diagnosis. Any eating regimen, including this one, should be undertaken only under the direct supervision of the reader's physician. In particular, this regimen should not be followed by anyone who has certain diseases or conditions, including, without limitation, diabetes, colitis, hypoglycemia, a spastic colon, ulcers, ileitis, enteritis, diverticulosis or by anyone who is pregnant or breast feeding. Moreover, anyone with other chronic or serious ailments or who is under treatment for a medical condition should undertake this eating program only under the direct supervision of his or her own physician.

Library of Congress Cataloging-in-Publication Data

Mazel, Judy.
    The new Beverly Hills diet recipes to forever : an eating book / Judy Mazel.
        p.   cm.
    Includes index.
    ISBN 1-55874-475-4 (pbk.)
    1. Reducing diets. 2. Food combining. I. Title.
RM222.2.M4313   1997
641.5'635—dc21   97-3323
                                             CIP

©1997 Judy Mazel and Michael Wyatt
ISBN 1-55874-475-4

Publisher: Health Communications, Inc.
              3201 S.W. 15th Street
              Deerfield Beach, FL 33442-8190

*To the "Eaters" of the world . . . those of you who,
like me, love to eat and live to eat; who, when food is
in your mouth, your heart sings and your soul soars:
I dedicate this book.*

*Eat your heart out . . . now you have your
recipe to forever!*

Contents

Golden Rules

1 Weigh yourself *every* day, no matter what.

2 FRUIT. Start almost every day of your life with fruit. Once you have eaten something other than fruit in the course of the day, never, never ever go back to eating fruit.

Fruit digests almost instantly. Before you can even finish eating a pineapple, its nutrients are being absorbed by your body. If it is inhibited in its digestion, if it is eaten after anything else, it gets trapped in your stomach by other foods. Its explosive enzyme action will be offset by bloating and gas. Your savior will be transformed into your torment.

3 THE WAITING TIME. When you go from one fruit to another fruit, wait one hour. When you go from one food group to another food group, wait two hours minimum (three would be better).

These are the minimum waiting times—the shortest periods of time you can get away with without running the risk of fat. Remember, you gain weight because food is not efficiently digested. In simpler terms, if food doesn't leave your stomach when it should, if it becomes trapped or held up by other antagonistic foods, the nutrients it should generate will not be properly processed by your body and you'll gain weight.

4 PROTEIN. Once you've eaten protein, even one little bite, at least 80 percent of what you eat for the remainder of the day should be protein.

Acknowledgments

It was a special blend of ingredients that turned this into such a tasty morsel. Thank you all for adding your own distinct flavor . . .

Nancy Marcantonio; Jean Brady; my mother; my sister, Carol; Roger Mouritson; David Henderson and Ellen Miley; IWT; Bob and Kathy Pearson; R&K Foods; Leslie Dillahunt and Harriet Kaufman; Lightning Corp.; Matthew Diener; and Margie and Herman Platt.

A special thanks to God and Gurus,
and Paramahansa Yogananda.

Introduction

Cooking and eating à la Conscious Combining isn't about deprivation, giving up or going without. It's also not about counting calories or grams of fat. And it's not about *anything* you've ever thought of as a "diet." It's about enjoying great food and using your good common sense. It's about living and having fun: a lifestyle eating plan that gets you thin and keeps you that way forever.

I repeat what I said throughout *The New Beverly Hills Diet*: YOU . . . WILL . . . NEVER . . . GO . . . WITHOUT! You will never go hungry. You will never have to give up your favorites. There are no "no's," no "never's" and no forbidden foods. You don't have to cheat to eat *anything*. One look at the selection of recipes and ingredients in this book should dispel any of your fears about self-denial. It's an eater's dream come true. Butter? You bet! Cream? As I said, it's all here!

You've found that pot of gold at the end of the rainbow: your chance to be as thin as you'd like for the rest of your life by simply taking charge of the food you eat. If you follow the few simple rules of Conscious Combining as explained in *The New Beverly Hills Diet* and effectively combine foods for optimum nutrition and slimhood, you will not only become a Born-Again Skinny, you will embrace healthful and joyful eating habits that will keep you slim *forever.*

An important part of taking charge of the food you eat is coming to terms with the *joy* food brings into our lives, not the sorrow. You now have permission to enjoy food: to experience it and make it an experience! All too often, "diets" fail to address the full range of our relationship with food. They recognize only the pain of being fat and make an obscenity out of loving to eat. *They are doomed to failure because they take all the joy out of eating.*

Food! Glorious food! It brings us sustenance. It brings us pleasure. It is the social force that binds people of diverse cultures together in the common wordless moment of a single delicious bite. Preparing food is more than a mundane daily task; it is an essential part of living—and should be a celebration of health, life and sharing! Whether you're dining out alone or feeding an army of family and friends at home, each time you eat should be an affirmation of well-being. Enjoy! Embrace the joy of food, but do it *consciously.* Select what you eat—and what you eat together—carefully. You can have it all—hamburgers and hipbones, cheesecake and cheekbones—if you only follow a simple handful of Conscious Combining rules.

As I said, *The New Beverly Hills Diet* is not about deprivation. And in the following pages I will prove it to you. You will not deny yourself food (or your love of it) in any way. Instead, we will look at food in all of its contexts. We'll run the gamut from the social focus of a party to meals on the run, from the healthful pleasures of a weekday family dinner to the luscious treasures of a gourmet feast. As we examine food in all these contexts, we will always have one thought in mind: the application of the principles of Conscious Combining.

Let your food fantasies run wild! Think of the following recipes as only a sampling, as a starting point for your own creative journey. Some of these recipes are easy. Others you may find challenging. So be adventurous in your eating—and in your cooking. When you dine out, try new dishes. Pick from the parts of the menu where you never dared venture before. Mix and match, pick and choose. Why not three appetizers and a dessert? Or four vegetables à la carte? And when you dine in, bring your adventures home. Try new ingredients and new cooking methods. Don't be shy about tackling a tough recipe or mixing styles and ingredients. Be bold! Have fun! If you just follow the rules of Conscious Combining, you'll never get in trouble.

The recipes in this book are certainly not intended to be an all-inclusive compilation. This is an *eating* book, not a cooking book. There is a world of taste treats out there waiting for you to discover and enjoy. I have assembled this collection to provide you with the foundation you need to prepare exciting and delectable foods that thrill the taste buds, delight the eye and yet adhere to the simple principles of Conscious Combining. It's up to you to go the next step by making these recipes and others you discover your own.

From everyday to elegant, these dishes offer you a

range of recipes that will fit any occasion. As you prepare these dishes, you will see how easy it is to convert any of your personal favorites as well as recipes from every cookbook on your shelf into healthful, Consciously Combined, nutritious and slim-friendly food.

So turn your kitchen into a temple of Conscious Combining! Throw out those artificial sweeteners! Toss your additive-packed "diet" foods and those low-fat, no-fat "healthy" choices. Keep that windowsill lined with pineapples, that fruit bowl filled, and stock your refrigerator and cupboards with fresh, whole foods. Start enjoying! As I said, you *can* have it all. Hamburgers and hipbones, cheesecake and cheekbones. You can be Born-Again Skinny forever!

COOKING CONSCIOUSLY

The effective application of Conscious Combining hinges on knowing not only what doesn't go together but *what goes together best*. These recipes illustrate some optimum combinations that will titillate your taste buds, maximize your energy and minimize your size. They are designed to feed your body as well as your heart and soul.

The Mazel Salad, for instance, with its wide variety of greens and its exciting mix of contrasting tastes and textures, is also rich in vitamins A and C, potassium, and calcium. With its snap of clear, fresh flavor, the LTO Salad is the perfect balance of flavor and nutrition.

If you have been following the eating plan of *The New Beverly Hills Diet* (If you haven't it's time to get started), you now welcome the fresh, clean taste of pure food. Flavors are opening up and growing more intense. You don't miss salt any longer, and you can probably tell when a sweetener made of chemicals has been added to your food or when it's "lite" mayonnaise instead of regular. Even the simplest foods now taste good, don't they? Sad, isn't it, how, other than Conscious Combiners, most people have no idea what a potato *really* tastes like? Or zucchini. Or pasta. You will find that using garlic and fresh spices like a pinch of grated ginger will enhance the flavor of almost anything.

Now that carbohydrates aren't something to fear, you might find that you much prefer your open-carb meals to open-protein meals. Then again, now that you have permission to eat dishes like fried calamari and barbecued spareribs, protein might still be your top pick. Whichever you prefer, go ahead. Enjoy! Find out for yourself.

If you're like most of us, many of your current favorite recipes combine proteins and carbs. If you experiment a little, you will find that the protein adds nothing to the flavor. It merely represents a different texture. If you omit it or substitute something else in the carb family for it, you probably won't miss it. The only thing you'll miss is the extra weight you would have put on from the indigestibility the protein brings to the carbs.

If you follow the rules and modify when you can, then you can eat all those glorious miscombinations (that are only glorious because they are miscombinations) when you want them. Remember: *If you think about food when it doesn't count, you don't have to think about it when it does.*

A big advantage to *The New Beverly Hills Diet* is that you don't have to prepare any special foods or cook in any new way. Almost any recipe can be adapted easily and flavorfully to Conscious Combining just by thinking about the rules and applying them.

So eat, enjoy and flaunt those hipbones! Skinny is now a forever reality because you have the *Recipes to Forever*!

Recipe Notes

SESAME OIL: Two types of sesame oil are available. Light oils are pressed from raw sesame seeds and are commonly found in health food stores and larger supermarkets. The second type—Asian-style amber-colored oils—are made from roasted sesame seeds and are used for flavor only. When assembling a recipe using sesame oil, check the instructions carefully to be sure you're using the type of sesame oil specified. Light and dark oils are not interchangeable. **The recipes in this book use light sesame oil for cooking.**

A MATTER OF TASTE: When I use the term "to taste" in the recipes, I mean exactly that. I try to be as specific as possible about the amounts of ingredients used, but tastes vary. For example, even if we all liked the same intensity of garlic (we don't!), garlic may differ in intensity from one variety or bulb to the next. For this reason, it is important to first be familiar with the distinctions among different varieties of ingredients. You should also know how long your finished product will sit before it is eaten (during which time the flavors will intensify accordingly). Then you can decide how much of a certain flavoring agent you wish to add. Of course, what you want to "star" in your dish may change with your mood. I, for one, like tons of garlic. For me, "too much" is never enough!

EATING FOR ONE: Just because you're cooking for one is no reason to limit your choice of recipes. Almost any dish can be scaled down for a single diner. All you have to do is reduce the ingredients according to the number of servings the recipe prepares. The exceptions are recipes with many ingredients and those with complex sauces. In these cases, make the entire recipe and freeze the remainder for a quick and easy meal another day. If you don't have it all today, you can have it tomorrow—it's not leaving the planet.

Editor's Note: When recipes included in this book appear as ingredients in other recipes, they are in boldface. Please check the index for the page numbers of ingredients appearing in boldface.

ONE

Sauces and Basics

Mazel Dressing

¹/₄ cup rice vinegar
1 cup light-colored
   sesame oil
Chopped garlic, to taste*
   (1 to 3 small cloves)

Chopped or grated ginger,
   to taste*
Freshly ground black pepper,
   to taste

Combine all ingredients.
YIELD: 1³/₄ cups

RICE VINEGAR: *Less pungent and more flavorful than distilled white vinegar, rice vinegar is available in three varieties: white, red and black. Red and black are commonly used for dipping sauces, while white is used for sweet-and-sour dishes and several recipes in this book.*

---

* From clove to clove and root to root, garlic and ginger may differ in intensity. If they are left to steep in dressing, their flavors will intensify. Therefore, depending on when you make the dressing, on the strength of the garlic and ginger, and, of course, on personal taste, the amounts used may differ. Start with 1 clove garlic and 6 to 7 gratings of ginger, and increase to up to 3 times that amount if desired.

Beurre Blanc
(White Butter Sauce)

Serve as a sauce with vegetables or alongside **Puff Pastry Tourte with Leek and Mushroom Filling** or **Spinach-Dill Tourte**. Delicious also with fish or shellfish.

4 tablespoons finely minced shallot
2 tablespoons rice vinegar (substitute stock or water when using with protein)

2 tablespoons water
1 tablespoon tepid water
4 ounces (1 stick) unsalted butter (room temperature), cut in pieces

Place shallot, vinegar and 2 tablespoons water in a small heavy saucepan and simmer over a low flame until all moisture evaporates and shallot is soft.

Remove from heat, add additional tablespoon water and whisk in the soft butter. (This is done off the heat so that the butter does not melt but begins to emulsify into a fluffy mass with the shallots.) When completed, sauce should have the consistency of a thick cream.

YIELD: 1 cup

Crème à l'Échalote
(Shallot Cream)

Delicious over poached fish, chicken or eggs.

2 tablespoons unsalted
  butter
4 tablespoons minced
  shallot
½ cup chicken or veal
  stock (**Fonds de
  Volaille** or **Fonds Brun**)
2 cups heavy cream

1 egg yolk
1 tablespoon fresh tarragon
  (or another herb
  appropriate to the use of
  the sauce; fennel or anise
  is a wonderful complement
  to fish)

Melt butter in a small heavy saucepan.

Add shallot and sauté until wilted and lightly browned.

Drain off butter and add chicken or veal stock; raise the heat and cook until the liquid is reduced by half.

Add the cream and cook over medium-high heat, whisking constantly, until the sauce is reduced by about one quarter.

Remove from heat and immediately add egg yolk and tarragon while whisking briskly. Serve warm.

YIELD: 2 cups

Béarnaise Sauce

Béarnaise is made by following the same simple technique used to make **Hollandaise Sauce**. It is, however, herb based, with more intense flavors.

2 tablespoons minced
  shallot
1 tablespoon fresh tarragon
  (or 2 teaspoons dried)
2 teaspoons dried chervil
2 tablespoons rice vinegar
  (or 2 tablespoons water or
  stock when using sauce
  with protein)

2 tablespoons water
Freshly ground white
  pepper, to taste
2 egg yolks
2 tablespoons water or
  stock
8 ounces (2 sticks)
  unsalted butter, melted

Place shallot, tarragon, chervil, vinegar, 2 table-spoons water and white pepper in a small heavy saucepan. Place over high heat and reduce until only 1 to 2 teaspoons of liquid remain. Add egg yolks and additional 2 tablespoons water or stock to the sauce. Whisk over low heat until thick and fluffy. Remove from heat.

Off heat, dribble in some of the melted butter and whisk constantly. Still whisking, slowly add the rest of the butter, taking care to omit the milky residue on the bottom. Whisk quickly so the sauce stays warm. The sauce should be thick and fluffy. Season with an additional pinch of white pepper and herbs, if desired.

YIELD: 2 cups

FRESH VERSUS DRIED HERBS: *As a general rule, use two to three times more fresh herbs than dried.*

Crème au Raifort
(Horseradish Cream)

Quick to make, this recipe adds great zip to all simply cooked beef dishes, from potted brisket to standing rib roast.

1 cup heavy cream
¼ cup freshly grated
* horseradish*
2 twists of freshly
* ground white pepper*

Pinch cayenne pepper
1 tablespoon whole
* green peppercorns*

Beat cream in a chilled bowl until stiff.

With the back of a spoon, press horseradish against a fine sieve to remove moisture. Combine horseradish with white pepper and cayenne.

Fold into whipped cream.

With a mortar and pestle, or simply with the bottom of a glass on a flat surface, crush the peppercorns and fold them into the whipped cream mixture.

Refrigerate until ready to serve.

YIELD: Approximately 1½ cups

Béchamel Sauce

A béchamel is a simple sauce to make, but a versatile one, with many uses. It can be a thickener for pureed vegetables and can be used as a base for creamed soups and sauces. Traditionally made by combining scalded milk with a roux of unsalted butter and flour, this Conscious-Combining recipe makes it with a thin roux, completing it with heavy cream.

2 cups heavy cream	*Grating of fresh nutmeg*
1 bay leaf	*2 tablespoons unsalted*
Twist of freshly ground	*butter*
white pepper	*2 tablespoons flour*

Heat cream in a heavy saucepan until it begins to bubble lightly at the edges. Remove from heat.

Add bay leaf, white pepper and nutmeg, cover, and set aside to steep.

Melt butter in a heavy saucepan until it bubbles.

Whisk in flour, making sure to incorporate thoroughly, and cook until it foams. Remove from heat until cooled somewhat.

Pour the cream over the butter and flour mixture (the roux), whisking constantly. Place the saucepan back on a medium flame and continue whisking until the sauce thickens. Cook over a low flame for 5 or 6 minutes more, whisking occasionally. Remove bay leaf.

If not used immediately, remove from heat and place a piece of plastic wrap directly on the surface of the sauce to prevent a skin from forming.

YIELD: Approximately 2 cups

Variation: Velouté

The velouté is the sister of the béchamel and is made exactly the same way except that vegetable stock is substituted for the cream; the butter and flour are increased to 3 tablespoons each; herbs are added, if desired; and cooking time is increased to 20 minutes. Skim off fat or impurities as it cooks. Lighter and less rich than a béchamel, a velouté is also used in purees and soups and as a sauce base.

COOKING TIMES: *The cooking times given are only suggestions because of the variables involved: the size of the pan, the way the pan heats, the temperature of the food, etc. Experimenting will be your best guide.*

Hollandaise Sauce

Hollandaise is a simple sauce to make. Once you get the hang of it, it should take you only about 3 to 5 minutes. Because it is categorized as a fat, it can be used to embellish either carbs or proteins.

2 egg yolks
2 tablespoons water
8 ounces (2 sticks)
unsalted butter, melted
and cooled slightly

Freshly ground white
pepper, to taste (optional)
Pinch of cayenne pepper
(optional)
Fresh chives, parsley and
tarragon (optional)

Place egg yolks and water in a heavy saucepan and begin whisking over a low flame. This will gently poach the egg in the water. You will feel it thicken as you whisk. When it has thickened, but before it begins to curdle or come apart, remove from heat.

Off heat, dribble in some of the melted butter, whisking constantly. Still whisking, slowly add the rest of the butter, taking care to omit the milky residue on the bottom. Whisk quickly so the sauce stays warm. The sauce should be thick and fluffy. Season with a twist of white pepper and cayenne and herbs, if desired.

You can warm the sauce very slightly over warm water for 1 or 2 minutes, but beware of heating too much—if overheated, the sauce will separate. If you have to hold the sauce, you may keep it over tepid water for a short while. Serve over vegetables, fish or eggs.

YIELD: 2 cups

Mazel Hollandaise Sauce*

1 tablespoon cold water
4 egg yolks
8 ounces (2 sticks)
   unsalted butter, cut into
   small pieces and at
   room temperature

1 tablespoon rice vinegar
Cayenne pepper to taste
Freshly ground black
   pepper, to taste

Beat water and egg yolks together over low heat** for a few seconds in a heavy pan. Then gradually add butter, raising and lowering pan so that the mixture does not get too hot. When all butter has emulsified (thoroughly combined with egg yolks), add vinegar and seasonings.

Pour mixture into a small thermos or hold over warm—not hot—water. Hollandaise does not need to be piping hot to be good; the food you're serving it on can be hot. If held over hot water, the hollandaise is very likely to separate. If this should happen, add a teaspoon or two of boiling water, whisk madly and pray!

YIELD: 2 cups

---

* This is classified as a fat and can be combined with a carbohydrate or a protein.

** Hollandaise is traditionally made in a double-boiler, which is fine if you are new at preparing the sauce. However, once you have learned to make it directly over the heat, you will find the cooking goes much faster.

Mazel Mayonnaise

You can make mayonnaise in a food processor or blender. It takes 2 to 8 minutes. Once you get into the habit, you will enjoy having fresh mayonnaise at hand for any number of uses.

Carb Mayonnaise

2 egg yolks
2 teaspoons rice vinegar
Freshly ground white
  pepper, to taste
1/4 teaspoon dry mustard

Pinch of cayenne pepper
1½ cups light-colored
  sesame oil

Place egg yolks, vinegar, white pepper, mustard and cayenne in a food processor or blender. Process or blend for 2 minutes.

With the processor or blender running, dribble the oil in. Proceed very slowly, adding only the smallest amount of oil until you see that the egg is absorbing the oil and a mayonnaise is forming. Then add the oil in a thin, steady stream.

Taste for seasonings. You may prefer to add more white pepper.

YIELD: 1½ cups

Protein Mayonnaise

1 whole egg
1 tablespoon stock or
   water
Freshly ground white
   pepper, to taste
$\frac{1}{4}$ teaspoon dry mustard

Pinch of cayenne pepper
$1\frac{1}{2}$ cups light-colored
   sesame oil

Place egg, stock or water, white pepper, mustard and cayenne in a food processor or blender. Process or blend for 2 minutes.

With the processor or blender running, dribble the oil in. Proceed very slowly, adding only the smallest amount of oil until you see that the egg is absorbing the oil and a mayonnaise is forming. Then add the oil in a thin, steady stream.

Taste for seasonings. You may prefer to add more white pepper.

YIELD: $1\frac{1}{2}$ cups

Variation 1: Mazel Herb Mayonnaise

Add chopped garlic, freshly ground white pepper or fresh herbs. If you are using a food processor and want to add herbs, chop them in the processor before making mayonnaise and blend them in at the last minute or leave them in while making mayonnaise to produce green mayonnaise (**Sauce Verte**). Good herb choices, depending on the season, are tarragon, basil, thyme, dill, parsley and chives. Use about $\frac{1}{4}$ cup chopped herbs per recipe if fresh, and 1 tablespoon if dried.

Variation 2: Sauce Verte (Green Mayonnaise)

Puree in a food processor or chop very fine: 1 bunch watercress (leaves only), 2 tablespoons chopped parsley and 1 tablespoon chopped fresh dill or tarragon. Fold into mayonnaise.

Variation 3: Mayonnaise aux Tomates (Tomato Mayonnaise)

Prepare 3 tomatoes by plunging into boiling water for 10 seconds, peeling and chopping. Push through a fine sieve to puree and remove seeds. Fold puree into mayonnaise for a thick tomato dressing.

Variation 4: Mayonnaise à la Moutarde (Mustard Mayonnaise)

Make a paste of 1 teaspoon dry mustard, 1 tablespoon mayonnaise and 1 tablespoon crushed green peppercorns. Fold paste into 1 cup mayonnaise.

Variation 5: Aïoli (Garlic Mayonnaise)

Mince 5 cloves of garlic and combine with ¼ cup mayonnaise in a food processor. Process until garlic is pureed into mayonnaise. Add a pinch of cayenne pepper and fold into 1 cup mayonnaise.

Pesto

While pesto is typically associated with a basil-based Italian sauce, other cuisines have their own versions of this herb-seasoning blend. You can use virtually any combination of your favorite herbs to make your own "signature" pesto.

Make pesto in the summer, when fresh herbs are most plentiful. Stored in airtight containers, pesto will stay fresh for up to two months in your refrigerator. To enjoy pesto all winter, place the finished sauce in small jars (do not fill completely) and store in the freezer. Or freeze the pesto in an ice-cube tray and wrap the individual cubes in plastic wrap. Individual taste for pesto is variable, though 2 to 3 tablespoons seems to be the norm. Each frozen cube of pesto is about 3 tablespoons, so each cube is enough for one serving (about 4 to 6 ounces of cooked pasta). In the freezer, pesto will remain good for up to six months.

Basic Basil Pesto

2 cups fresh basil leaves,   4 cloves garlic, minced
   stems removed, tightly   Olive oil
   packed

Wash and dry basil leaves thoroughly. Place leaves
in bowl of food processor. Add garlic; process until
basil and garlic are chopped and combined.

Dribble in olive oil through feed tube. Take care to
add only enough to make pesto thick and pasty.

YIELD: ³/₄ cup

Pesto for Pasta

½ cup parsley (preferably
  Italian) stems removed
¾ cup fresh basil leaves,
  stems removed, tightly
  packed
4 cloves garlic, peeled
  and trimmed

½ cup olive oil
Freshly ground black
  pepper, to taste
Liquid in which pasta was
  cooked (sufficient amount
  for thinning pesto to
  sauce consistency)

Puree first three ingredients with mortar and pestle, or in food processor or blender. Dribble in olive oil until pesto is thick and pasty. Season with pepper. Whisk reserved liquid into pesto and toss pesto with pasta.

YIELD: ¾ cup

Marinara Sauce

Make marinara in the summer, when tomatoes are luscious. Freeze for use all winter.

7 tablespoons olive oil	*10 leaves fresh basil*
2 onions, chopped	*1 sprig fresh oregano*
4 cloves garlic, minced	*1 sprig fresh thyme*
4 pounds tomatoes,	*Freshly ground black*
seeded and chopped	*pepper, to taste*

Heat the oil in a large heavy saucepan. Add onions and cook slowly until wilted (about 15 minutes), but do not brown. Add garlic and tomatoes; toss with oil and onion in pan. Add herbs and pepper, cover, and cook until tomatoes are soft and flavors are blended (approximately ½ hour). Cool for 5 minutes.

Place sauce in a food processor or blender and lightly puree the sauce with on/off chopping motion. Sauce may be frozen for later use.

YIELD: 6 to 8 cups (depending on variety of tomatoes)

Mazel Marinara

1 cup finely chopped onion
4 teaspoons olive oil
½ cup finely chopped
 carrot
2 teaspoons fresh basil
 or **Basic Basil Pesto**
4 teaspoons finely
 chopped parsley

½ bay leaf
2 pounds fresh tomatoes,
 coarsely chopped*
1 tablespoon tomato paste
 (salt-free, of course)
Freshly ground black
 pepper, to taste
Red pepper flakes, to taste
 (optional)

Cook onion in oil until translucent. Add carrot and cook 4 minutes. Add basil or pesto, parsley and bay leaf; simmer 2 minutes. Add tomatoes, tomato paste and pepper; simmer 30 minutes. Add red pepper flakes, if desired.

YIELD: 3 cups

---

* You may want to peel tomatoes for some dishes, such as pizza, as the peels definitely change the texture of the dish.

Sauce Rouille

1 egg yolk
2 tablespoons chopped
  garlic
¹/₄ teaspoon paprika
¹/₂ teaspoon fish stock
  or **Fumet de Poisson**

¹/₄ teaspoon cayenne
Freshly ground black
  pepper, to taste
1 cup olive oil

Place all ingredients, excluding oil, in a food processor and process for 1 minute. Dribble oil into yolk mixture and continue to process until sauce is thickened.

YIELD: 1¹/₄ cups or 4 to 5 servings

Mazel Ketchup

1 pound plum tomatoes
1 small onion, minced
1/4 teaspoon cayenne pepper
1 clove garlic

1 teaspoon dried oregano
Freshly ground black
  pepper, to taste

In a large pot of boiling water, cook tomatoes for 3 minutes, just until softened. Drain immediately and plunge into a bowl of cold water.

Peel, seed and dice tomatoes.

Place tomatoes and remaining ingredients in a food processor or blender and puree.

YIELD: Approximately 1 cup

Mazel "Cheese," Mexican or Italian

ॐ

6 onions, peeled and
  thinly sliced
¼ to ½ cup corn or
  olive oil (corn oil for
  Mexican, olive oil for
  Italian)
1 to 2 cloves garlic,
  minced

½ cup chopped cilantro
  (for Mexican)
¼ teaspoon dried oregano
  (for Italian)
1 teaspoon chopped fresh
  thyme or ¼ teaspoon
  dried thyme (for Italian)

Cook onions in ¼ cup oil, adding more oil if onions
start to stick to pan and dry out. Cook until soft and
cheeselike. If using medium heat, stop cooking after
20 minutes; on low heat, continue cooking for 45
minutes or longer, stirring every few minutes and
being careful not to burn.

For Mazel Cheese Mexican, add garlic and cilantro
at end of cooking time.

For Mazel Cheese Italian, add garlic, oregano and
thyme at end of cooking time.

YIELD: 3 cups

Hot and Spicy Salsa Mazel

1 large onion
2 tablespoons corn oil
6 cloves garlic, minced
2 to 6 fresh New Mexico
  chili peppers, minced
2 fresh jalapeño peppers,
  minced (optional—eliminate
  to make it less hot)

8 large tomatoes, chopped
2 tablespoons chopped
  fresh parsley
2 tablespoons chopped
  fresh cilantro

As a precaution, wear gloves when handling chili peppers and avoid touching your eyes. These peppers are hot little devils.

Mince onion and sauté in oil for 3 to 4 minutes. Soften but do not brown.

Add garlic to onions. Add chili and jalapeño peppers. (If fresh chilies are not available, substitute 2 tablespoons dry red chili powder.) Sauté mixture an additional 1 to 2 minutes, but do not brown.

Add tomatoes and sauté 5 minutes or until salsa is desired thickness.

Take off heat. Add parsley and cilantro.

YIELD: Approximately 2 cups (the longer you cook it, the smaller the amount and the hotter it will be)

Note: The smaller the chili, the hotter the taste.

HOT STUFF: *The New World contributed many delights to the world's cuisine, including the Aztec* tomatl *(the tomato) and* xocoatl *(chocolate), as well as corn, vanilla, papayas, pumpkins and peanuts. But none is greater than the chili.*

Fresh Mexican Salsa

8 large tomatoes, coarsely
  diced
1 large onion, chopped
2 cloves garlic, minced
2 tablespoons chopped
  fresh parsley

2 tablepoons coarsely
  chopped fresh cilantro
1/4 to 2 teaspoons grated
  jalapeño pepper*

Combine all ingredients and mix thoroughly.
YIELD: 5 cups

CHILIES: *Chilies have been a part of the Mesoamerican menu for over 7,000 years. Wild chilies—peanut-size and very, very hot—originated in what is now Bolivia and eventually spread throughout South and Central America.*

---

* To make handling jalapeños easier (and less hazardous!), freeze them before grating.

Tomatillo Salsa

1 pound fresh tomatillos,
  husks removed
¼ cup chopped cilantro
1 teaspoon grated or finely
  minced jalapeño pepper
1 yellow onion, chopped

2 cloves garlic, minced
1 teaspoon ground cumin
½ teaspoon ground
  coriander
1 teaspoon **Powdered
  Chilies**

Core tomatillos, chop very fine and place in medium-size mixing bowl. Add cilantro, jalapeño pepper, onion, garlic and spices. Mix to combine. Cover and refrigerate for at least an hour.

YIELD: Approximately 2 cups

POWDERED CHILIES: *Don't buy chili powder—it is a mix of several ingredients, including cumin, oregano and salt. Make your own flavorful mix instead. Choose among the many varieties of dried chilies available at most large supermarkets or specialty food stores. My favorite is a mix of poblano and chipotle chilies—they have a wonderful smoky flavor with a delightful heat!*

The best tool for grinding chilies (and other herbs and spices) is a coffee grinder. Typically available for under $25, these small grinders are a handy addition to any kitchen. To grind, cut the chilies into pieces small enough to fit into the grinder. Experience is the best guide to grinding times. You'll soon find out how long it takes to grind the chilies to the size you prefer. After grinding, place in an airtight container to preserve freshness.

Any-Fruit Frozen Puree

Here's a refreshing change of pace for fruit (and a great treat on those dog days of summer). Remember, use only one fruit at a time in the recipes, and wait at least one hour before switching from eating one fruit to eating another.

2 pounds any fruit—pineapple, papaya, strawberries, grapes, etc.

Wash and dry fruit. Peel, if necessary, and slice into chunks that will fit easily into your food processor or blender. Blend or process adding water as needed. Make the puree smooth or chunky depending on what you like.

Pour pureed mixture into ice cube trays or paper cups, nonstick muffin tins, etc. Cover with plastic wrap. (Poke a popsicle stick through the plastic wrap on the paper cups before freezing, and you've made a refreshing frozen-fruit puree bar.) Freeze 2 to 3 hours or until firm.

To serve, place frozen fruit cubes into your blender or processor and process until smooth. Serve immediately.

YIELD: Variable

No-Salt Quick Dill Pickles

∽

3 sprigs fresh dill
1½ tablespoons mustard
    seed
2 tablespoons whole
    allspice
6 cloves garlic, peeled

3½ pounds 3- to 4-inch
    unwaxed pickling
    cucumbers
1 quart rice vinegar*
1 quart water

When making pickles it is imperative that you use the freshest cucumbers you can find.

Begin by washing 6 wide-mouth pint canning jars in hot, soapy water. Make sure that none are cracked and that the mouths are smooth and free of nicks. Rinse well. Prepare new canning lids per manufacturer's directions.

In each jar place ½ head of a dill sprig, ¼ tablespoon mustard seed, ⅓ tablespoon whole allspice and 1 clove garlic, halved. Garlic can be increased to taste.

Wash cucumbers in fresh water and drain. Cut lengthwise into quarters. Pack quarters vertically into canning jars, making sure to trim them so that there is ½ inch of headroom at the top of each jar. Do not force too many cucumbers into the jars. If you pack the jars too tightly, the cucumbers will not pickle evenly.

In a 2- to 3-quart glass container, combine vinegar and water. Pour mixture over cucumbers in jars,

---

* Rice vinegar must have five percent acidity, so check several brands.

being careful to leave $^1/_2$ inch of space at the top. Run a table knife around the inside of the jars to release any trapped air. Wipe rims with a clean dishtowel. Set lids on jars and tighten bands to hand-tight—do not overtighten.

Place a rack at the bottom of a large stockpot or canner and fill pot two-thirds full of water. Bring to a boil and reduce to simmer. Place jars in water, making sure water level is at least 1 inch higher than tops of the jars. When the water temperature reaches 180°F, process pickles uncovered for 20 minutes. Do not cover pan with lid. Using a jar lifter and without tilting the jars (tilting can break the seal), lift processed pickles out of water. Set jars on a towel and allow to cool. Check lids by pressing down on the centers; if they remain down, the jars are sealed properly.

Store sealed pickles for up to 2 years in a cool, dark place.

YIELD: 6 pints

T W O

Special
Seasonings

Once you are committed to Conscious Combining with the ultimate in elegant and healthful foods, your search will begin for delicious and exciting new ways to season your carbs and proteins.

The easiest and most delicious way I've discovered is through the flavor-filled glories of herbs and spices. The list of possibilities is almost endless: tarragon, thyme, oregano, sage, basil, savory, ginger, marjoram, cardamom, dill, fennel, anise, coriander, sorrel, cayenne, peppercorns (black, white or green) . . . and more! All will impart wonderful flavors to your cooking. Try growing your own herbs in summer. They flourish easily—the bugs don't like them as much as you will! Dry or freeze them to use all winter. Use them to make herb vinegars, piquant mustards or herb butters.

Herb Vinegar

2 cups rice vinegar   *1 bunch fresh herbs*

Bring rice vinegar to a boil. Pour over fresh herbs (for example, tarragon, oregano, garlic, rosemary or thyme) in a glass jar. Cover and allow to steep in a warm spot for at least two weeks. Strain to remove herbs, replace with a fresh sprig, cover and label. Use in salads and sauces.

YIELD: Approximately 2 cups

Mustard

You can turn dry mustard into a delicious condiment.

¹/₄ cup dry mustard
1 tablespoon rice vinegar
* (carbohydrate), or*
* 1 tablespoon water or*
* stock (protein)*
1 tablespoon minced herbs

1 clove garlic, minced
2 teaspoons minced
* shallot*
Freshly ground black
* pepper or crushed green*
* peppercorns, to taste*

Place mustard in a small mixing bowl. Combine with rice vinegar (or water or stock), herbs of your choice, garlic, shallot and pepper or peppercorns. The result should approximate the consistency of ordinary mustard.

YIELD: ¹/₄ cup

Herb Butter

½ cup butter, softened	Pinch of cayenne pepper
2 to 3 tablespoons minced herbs	Freshly ground black pepper, to taste (optional)
1 teaspoon minced garlic	

Blend butter, your favorite herb (parsley, chives, dill, tarragon, thyme or savory, all work well), garlic and cayenne. Add pepper, if desired.

Next, spread the butter-herb mixture in a thick line onto a piece of plastic wrap. Tightly close the plastic wrap around the mixture and shape into a "log." Twist the two open ends of the wrap shut. Place in the refrigerator until ready to use (wait at least two hours for flavor to develop) or freeze for later use (within 6 weeks). To add a flavorful punch to recipes, cut off slices of butter as needed.

Use to top grilled or poached fish, chicken, beef, lamb or vegetables. Spread under skin of chicken or fish when grilling or use as a final enrichment in soups.

YIELD: Approximately ½ cup

Garlic Butter

3 cloves garlic, mashed   *¹/₂ cup butter, softened*

Blend garlic into butter. Use over grilled steak or chops.

YIELD: Approximately ¹/₂ cup

Pimento Butter

1 red bell pepper　　　　　　*½ cup butter, softened*

Char, peel, seed and chop pepper, and mash into a smooth paste; blend in butter. Use on pasta or with fresh vegetables.

YIELD: Approximately ½ cup

Mel's Secret Seasoning

1 jalapeño pepper   *2 tablespoons olive oil*

Char, peel, seed and chop jalapeño pepper. Place in a shallow pan on medium heat with oil. Sauté until softened. Store in a jar and use when you want to add real zing to any sauce or vegetable.

YIELD: A few tablespoons

THREE

❦

Appetizers

Steamed Artichokes Stuffed with Tabbouleh

Rice vinegar	*2 artichokes*
Peppercorns	*1 recipe Couscous Mazel*
Basil	*1/2 red bell pepper, cored*
Oregano	*and diced*

In a large stock pot or pasta cooker place a steamer basket. Fill with water until it just comes to the bottom of the basket. Add rice vinegar, peppercorns, basil and oregano. Trim base of artichoke (stem) flat. Place artichokes stem up on steamer basket. Bring to boil over high heat, then reduce heat and simmer for 45 minutes or until tender and leaves remove easily. Cool until easy to handle, then use a spoon to scoop out the choke. Be careful not to scoop out the heart (that's the best part!)

Stuff cooled and hollowed artichokes with Couscous Mazel. Garnish with diced red peppers.

YIELD: 2 servings

Roasted Vegetable Medley

2 small zucchini
2 sweet onions
1 red bell pepper
1½ pounds small red
  potatoes

3 tablespoons sesame oil
1 teaspoon dried thyme
1 teaspoon dried basil
1 teaspoon dried oregano
1 teaspoon dried rosemary

Preheat oven to 425°F.

Scrub all vegetables and allow to dry thoroughly. Cut zucchini into 1- to 2-inch pieces, depending on diameter. Slice onions into bite-size wedges. Cut red pepper into 1-inch-wide strips. Cut any large potatoes in half.

In a bowl, combine oil and herbs. Whisk to mix thoroughly. Coat all vegetables with oil-herb mixture and arrange in a single layer in a 9 x 13-inch baking dish. Bake for 20 minutes or until vegetables are tender and lightly browned.

YIELD: 4 servings

Shrimp, Egg and Avocado Salad

2 cups cooked chicken,
  chopped
1 recipe **Garlic Aïoli** made
  with **Protein Mayonnaise**
4 hard boiled eggs, chilled

1½ pounds medium
  shrimp, cooked with
  heads, tails and shells
  removed
2 tablespoons slivered
  almonds

Place cooked chicken in a small bowl and combine with aïoli. Cut eggs into 8 wedges and set aside.

On four salad plates, arrange eggs and shrimp in a circular pattern. Place ¼ of the chicken aïoli mixture in the middle of each plate. Garnish with slivered almonds.

YIELD: 4 servings

Eggplant Dip

1 medium eggplant (approximately ³/₄ to 1 pound)
1 large yellow onion
2 tablespoons sesame oil
1 teaspoon red chili paste,
   or to taste
3 cloves garlic, pressed

Rice vinegar
Vegetable Stock, as
   needed
2 tablespoons chopped
   parsley
Green onions, sliced, for
   garnish

Cut eggplant in half lengthwise. Place cut side down on a baking sheet lined with foil. Place under hot broiler for about 15 minutes or until pulp is soft and skin blisters. Remove from oven and allow to cool.

While eggplant is broiling, slice onion into thin slices and sauté with sesame oil until soft and caramelized. Allow to cool.

When eggplant is cool enough to handle, scoop pulp out with a spoon. The remaining eggplant shell makes an interesting serving dish for this dip, so scoop carefully. Into the bowl of a food processor, add eggplant, onion, chili paste, garlic and rice vinegar. Begin to process slowly adding stock as needed to create a smooth consistency. Place dip into a small bowl, add parsley and mix well by hand. Garnish with sliced green onion. Serve at room temperature.

YIELD: Approximately 2¹/₂ cups

Shrimp and Scallop Skewers

1½ pounds large shrimp,
  in the shell
1½ pounds sea scallops
2 cloves garlic, finely
  minced or pressed

1 tablespoon grated ginger
1 teaspoon sesame oil
  (amber-colored, Asian-
  style)
Toasted sesame seeds

You will need 8-inch bamboo skewers.

Peel and devein shrimp. Rinse shrimp and scallops with cold water and pat dry with paper towels.

Preheat oven on broil. Combine all other ingredients except sesame seeds in a large bowl. Add shrimp and scallops to mixture; coat thoroughly.

Arrange seafood on skewers and broil under high heat for 5 minutes, turning once. Sprinkle with toasted sesame seeds and serve.

YIELD: 4 to 6 servings

Sesame-Coriander Shrimp

2 tablespoons sesame oil
(amber-colored, Asian-
style)
2 tablespoons ground
coriander
1 teaspoon ground black
pepper

1½ pounds large shrimp,
in the shell
2 tablespoons roasted
sesame seeds

In a large bowl, combine sesame oil, coriander and black pepper to make a marinade; set aside.

Peel and devein shrimp. Rinse shrimp with cold water and dry with a paper towel. Coat shrimp thoroughly with marinade, cover and allow to stand refrigerated for 30 minutes. Preheat broiler; broil shrimp until done, 4 to 6 minutes. Sprinkle with roasted sesame seeds and serve.

YIELD: 2 to 3 servings

Caramelized Garlic Toasts

¹/₄ cup olive oil
3 large heads garlic
1 sourdough baguette

4 tablespoons unsalted
  butter

Pour oil into an 8 x 8-inch glass baking dish. Cut the tops off the garlic heads, and place cut-side down in the oiled baking dish. Bake in 350°F. oven for about 1 hour or until inner cloves are soft and light brown. Remove from oven and allow to cool.

While garlic is roasting, slice baguette into ¹/₂-inch rounds and butter one side. Place buttered side down in a nonstick pan and fry until golden brown. Drain on paper towel.

Remove roasted garlic cloves from husks and place in a small bowl. Mash thoroughly. Spread mashed garlic on buttered side of toasts and place toasts on baking sheet.

Place baking sheet under preheated broiler and broil until golden brown. Serve alone as an appetizer or as a tasty addition to vegetable soup.

YIELD: Variable

Spicy Peppered Tuna Strips

4 yellowfin tuna steaks
(4 to 5 ounces each)
2 teaspoons sesame oil
4 tablespoons cracked
green peppercorns

*2 tablespoons **Powdered***
Chilies

Rinse tuna steaks and pat dry with a paper towel. Coat tuna steaks with sesame oil. Sprinkle tuna steaks liberally with cracked peppercorns and powdered chilies.

Heat nonstick pan on high heat. When hot, add tuna and quickly sear the steaks on each side—no more than 1 to 2 minutes per side.

Remove from pan and quickly cut tuna steaks into $1/2$-inch-thick strips. Place with cut side up for best appearance.

YIELD: 4 servings

FOUR

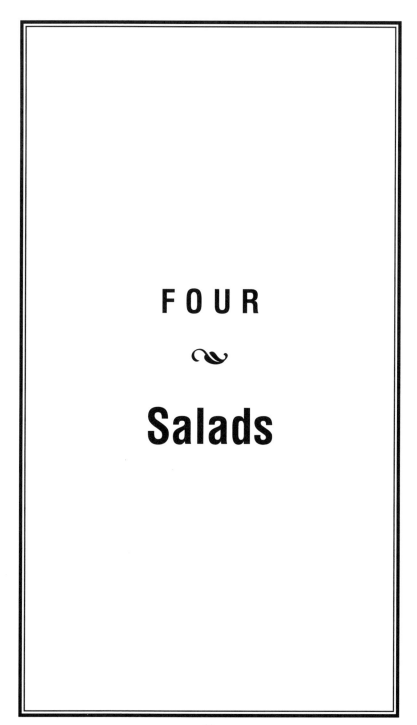

Salads

Salads can be a refreshing mainstay of a carbohydrate meal. Few dishes can compare to the healthful, delicious crunch of fresh greens or the flavorful, filling pleasure of chilled pasta and garden vegetables.

You'll find an increasing variety of greens available at many markets—often packaged already trimmed and washed. Don't be shy about substituting something new!

To make your salad as healthful and pleasurable as possible, be sure to wash salad greens thoroughly to remove any sand, grit or chemical residue. Wash the greens in several stages, using cold running water. Dressing won't adhere to wet greens so be sure to dry the greens well. You can use a salad spinner or just place them on paper towels, arranging greens and towels in alternating layers.

Note that greens start wilting as soon as they're tossed with a dressing. For the best texture and fullest flavor, be sure to add the dressing just before serving.

Mazel Salad

2 bunches spinach
2 bunches watercress
2 small heads Belgian
  endive
1 to 2 bunches mustard
  greens
3 carrots, grated

2 raw beets, grated
1 daikon radish, grated
25 mushrooms, cleaned
  and sliced
1 bunch chopped parsley
3 leeks cut on diagonal
  in ¼-inch pieces
Mazel Dressing

Be sure all vegetables are clean and thoroughly dry. Tear spinach, watercress, endive and mustard greens into large, bite-size pieces. Toss all ingredients with Mazel Dressing.

YIELD: 2 servings

VEGETABLES: *All vegetables should be fresh and of the finest quality. Rinse all vegetables carefully. When sautéing or stir-frying, excess water causes vegetables to steam, so be sure to dry them thoroughly. They should also be dried if tossed uncooked with egg-yolk-only mayonnaise or dressing—the water will dilute and make the dressing runny.*

Mazel Slaw

1 large green cabbage,
   grated
4 carrots, grated
1 bunch scallions, sliced
   diagonally

Carb Mayonnaise
   (egg-yolk-only) or
Mazel Dressing

Combine vegetables. Toss gently with desired dressing to serve.

YIELD: 2 servings

Mini-Mazel

2 bunches spinach,
   washed thoroughly
20 mushrooms, cleaned
   and sliced

3 to 4 large leeks, cleaned
   and trimmed carefully
Mazel Dressing

Combine vegetables. Toss with dressing to serve.
YIELD: 2 servings

LTO Salad

1 large, firm head
  iceberg lettuce
4 tomatoes
1 to 2 cucumbers, peeled

1 large red or Spanish
  onion, peeled
Mazel Dressing or
  olive oil

With a sharp knife, cut all vegetables into good-size chunks. Toss with desired dressing to serve.

YIELD: 2 servings

Sweet 'n' Sour Salad

A great combination of sweet basil and tangy watercress leaves.

2 cups basil leaves,
   washed, dried and
   chopped
2 bunches watercress
   leaves and tender tops
   of stems, washed, dried
   and chopped

3 large tomatoes (or 4
   medium), chopped into
   large chunks
2 cups chopped onion
3 cloves garlic, chopped
$\frac{1}{2}$ cup olive oil,
   approximately

In a large salad bowl, combine basil, watercress, tomatoes and onion.

Sprinkle the chopped garlic over all, then toss with olive oil. Use only enough oil to lightly coat the salad. Do not saturate or the salad will wilt.

YIELD: 2 servings

Insalata di Pasta
(Pasta Salad)

3 tablespoons olive oil
1 pound small shells,
  bow ties or rotelle
  (corkscrew-shaped pasta)
½ bunch broccoli
½ head cauliflower
10 asparagus tips
½ pound snow peas
2 red bell peppers
1 green bell pepper

⅓ cup heavy cream,
  approximately
1 cup **Mazel Mayonnaise**,
1 cup **Aïoli**,
  or ½ cup **Aïoli** mixed with
  ½ cup **Pesto for Pasta**
Herbs of your choice: thyme,
  basil, etc. (preferably fresh)
Freshly ground black
  pepper, to taste

In a large pot of boiling water, add 1 tablespoon olive oil and cook pasta until just firm, or al dente. Drain immediately. Rinse in cold water. Toss with 2 tablespoons oil in a large bowl. Set aside to cool.

Cut broccoli and cauliflower into florets and parboil. You want them to remain crisp, so be careful not to overcook them—2 to 3 minutes should be sufficient if the florets are small enough. Drain and refresh under cold water. Cook asparagus tips the same way; refresh (rinse under cold water). The snow peas will need only about 15 seconds of cooking; refresh immediately. Place red and green peppers under the broiler, char them on all sides and peel off the skin. Cut into strips.

Bit by bit, whisk heavy cream into mayonnaise to thin it sufficiently so that it will coat pasta. You may not need all the cream, depending on the consistency of your mayonnaise.

Combine pasta and vegetables. Toss with
mayonnaise-cream mixture and coat thoroughly.
Add herbs, grind black pepper over all and toss. Chill
and serve.

YIELD: 4 servings

Asian Watercress and Sprout Salad

1 pound watercress
1 pound mung-bean
  sprouts
2 bunches green onions
2 tablespoons Asian-style
  sesame oil
1/2 teaspoon freshly ground
  black pepper, or to taste

1 teaspoon rice vinegar
2 cloves garlic, minced or
  pressed
2 teaspoons grated fresh
  ginger
1 teaspoon red pepper
  sauce

Remove stems from watercress and discard. Rinse leaves thoroughly and drain in colander.

Fill a large pot with 2 quarts of water. Bring to a boil and add watercress and sprouts. Quickly mix to cover with water. After 30 seconds, remove from heat, place in colander and rinse immediately with cold running water. Allow to drain and cool, then squeeze gently to remove any remaining water.

Loosen clumps of watercress and sprouts and place in large bowl. Rinse green onions, remove tip with roots and about 2 inches of green tops; chop remainder into 1/4-inch slices. Add green onions and remaining ingredients to bowl. Toss to combine thoroughly, refrigerate and serve.

YIELD: 4 servings

Green Bean, Asparagus and Radish Salad

1½ cups rice vinegar
1½ cups water
1 medium red onion
½ pound green beans

½ pound asparagus
1 small daikon radish
½ pound whole cherry
  tomatoes

Dressing:
  ½ cup sesame oil
  ½ cup rice vinegar
  1 clove garlic, crushed
  2 tablespoons Dijon
    mustard

  ½ teaspoon oregano
  ½ teaspoon basil
  ½ teaspoon black pepper

Put tea kettle on to boil. Combine rice vinegar and water in a medium sized bowl; stir and set aside. Peel onion and slice into very thin slivers. Rinse beans and cut in julienne strips. Rinse asparagus and cut into 2-inch pieces. If stems are tough, discard them and use only tender ends.

Place beans, asparagus and onions into a colander and place in kitchen sink. When water boils, pour slowly over vegetables in colander; drain well. Place vegetables in marinade. Allow to marinate at room temperature for 1 to 2 hours.

Peel radish and cut into julienne strips. Rinse and dry tomatoes; remove stems. If tomatoes are large, halve them.

In a large salad bowl combine marinated vegetables, radish and tomatoes. Add about $\frac{1}{2}$ of the dressing and toss gently to coat. Serve remaining dressing on the side.

YIELD: 4 servings

Zucchini, Broccoli and Jicama Slaw

½ cup **Carb Mayonnaise**
1 tablespoon rice vinegar
½ small yellow onion,
  grated
1 teaspoon sugar
1 teaspoon caraway seed

¼ teaspoon white pepper
2 medium zucchini, grated
4 broccoli stems, grated
1 small jicama, peeled and
  diced
1 head butter or bib lettuce

In a small bowl combine mayonnaise, vinegar, yellow onion, sugar, caraway seed and white pepper. Mix well.

In a medium bowl combine zucchini, broccoli and jicama. Add dressing and mix until well coated. Cover and chill for 2 hours.

Serve on crisp butter lettuce leaves.

YIELD: 4 servings

FIVE

Soups on the Carb Side

For generations, soups have confidently held center stage in nearly every cuisine. Hearty and filling or light and refreshing, soups are the food of warmth, comfort and hospitality. Traditionally, they express the character of the culture and the range of ingredients available where they were first developed. What is more French than bouillabaisse or more reminiscent of a foggy Northeastern shore than chowder?

Here is a selection of soups for every occasion—but they are only a beginning. If you love soup as I do, you'll be pleased to know that soup is one of the most adaptable dishes in the Conscious-Combining menu. With only a few changes, it is likely that your favorite soup recipe can be converted to your new slim lifestyle.

Vegetable Stock

6 onions	5 scallions
2 carrots	1 large bunch parsley
4 leeks	Vegetable scraps saved
10 celery stalks with	during the week
leaves	1 tablespoon unsalted
3 parsnips	butter
3 tomatoes	5 quarts water
10 mushrooms	

Preheat oven to 350°F.

Wash and slice vegetables and parsley. Melt butter and combine with the vegetables. Turn into large casserole.

Bake, uncovered, for 30 minutes. Remove from oven. Add 5 quarts of water to casserole, partially cover and simmer on top of stove for 4 hours. Strain and refrigerate or freeze.

YIELD: 4 quarts

MUSHROOMS: *Clean mushrooms by wiping them with a paper towel or by washing them with a little water. If you use water, dry the mushrooms immediately with a paper towel or they may become soggy.*

Potage Crème de Légume
(Cream of Vegetable Soup)

Starting with a béchamel base, add a pureed vegetable, herbs and spices to create any number of creamed vegetable soups.

YIELD: 4 servings

Variation 1: Potage Crème de Choux Brocolis (Cream of Broccoli Soup)

Wash and coarsely dice 1 large bunch of broccoli. Cook in boiling water until fork-tender. Drain and puree in food processor or blender. Add puree to 2 cups heated **Velouté**, whisking to combine thoroughly. Season with freshly ground pepper, nutmeg and oregano and thyme to taste. Thin to desired consistency with heavy cream.

Variation 2: Potage Crème de Céleri (Cream of Celery Soup)

Wash and dice 1 head of celery, including leaves. Cook in boiling water until tender. Drain and puree in food processor or blender. Season with freshly ground white pepper, nutmeg, cayenne, marjoram and sage to taste. Add puree to 2 cups **Velouté**, whisking thoroughly. Heat through and thin with 1/2 cup heavy cream if desired.

Variation 3: Potage Crème Nivernaise
(Cream of Carrot Soup)

Wash, peel and slice 1 pound of carrots into $1/4$-inch rounds. Boil until fork-tender, drain and puree in food processor or blender. Season with freshly ground pepper, nutmeg, 2 tablespoons fresh thyme and a pinch of cayenne. Add puree to 2 cups **Velouté**, whisking thoroughly. Thin with heavy cream to desired consistency.

Variation 4: Potage à la Florentine
(Cream of Spinach Soup)

Follow instructions for **Potage Crème de Choux Brocolis**, substituting spinach for broccoli. Puree spinach with 1 clove of minced garlic, if desired, and season with dill, nutmeg and pepper.

Variation 5: Potage aux Navets
(Cream of Turnip Soup)

Follow instructions for **Potage Crème Nivernaise**, substituting turnips for carrots.

Potage Parmentier
(Leek and Potato Soup)

∾

4 medium leeks	6 cups water
2 tablespoons unsalted butter	Freshly ground white pepper, to taste
6 boiling potatoes (about 1½ pounds)	Sprig of fresh thyme
2 tablespoons flour	½ cup heavy cream
	Sour cream (optional)

Trim leeks to within an inch of the white part and discard the green. Cut a shallow cross in the stem end and wash leeks thoroughly under a strong stream of cold water, making sure to get all the sand out. Slice leeks into thin rounds.

Melt butter in a saucepan, stir in leeks and cook over low heat until leeks are wilted. Do not brown them. While leeks are cooking, wash and peel potatoes; slice thinly.

Whisk flour into leeks and butter, and cook until absorbed but not browned.

Boil water. Add water slowly to the leek mixture, whisking to be certain flour is absorbed. Add potatoes, pepper and thyme. Cover and simmer just until potatoes are tender.

Puree in a food processor or put through a food mill, reheat and add cream.

Spoon into serving bowls and, if desired, garnish with a dollop of sour cream.

YIELD: 6 servings

LEEKS: *Leeks are loosely structured, and they must be cleaned carefully. Slit them open and clean every layer separately. Grit is not a sensual texture.*

Corn Chowder

3 tablespoons unsalted butter	2 cups fresh corn kernels (frozen if fresh is unavailable)
1 onion, peeled and sliced	
2 boiling potatoes, peeled and cubed	2 tablespoons flour
2½ cups water	¼ cup water
Bouquet garni of parsley, bay leaf, fresh thyme and celery stalk with leaves, tied together with string or wrapped in a square of cheesecloth	1 cup heavy cream
	2 egg yolks

Melt butter in a large saucepan. Wilt onion in butter; add potatoes, 2½ cups water and bouquet garni. Cover and simmer gently for 15 minutes.

Add corn to soup mixture and cook until vegetables are fork-tender.

Blend flour into ¼ cup water with a small whisk. Add to soup mixture and stir to dissolve. Whisk in cream and simmer over medium heat until soup thickens.

In a small bowl, whisk egg yolks until thickened and sticky. By spoonfuls, beat about ¾ cup of the soup into egg yolks.

Remove bouquet garni from soup pot, stir mixture of egg yolks and soup back into larger pot. Do not allow to boil or egg will curdle. Serve immediately.

YIELD: 4 servings

Borscht

8 small to medium beets
 (the smaller the beet, the
 more intense the color
 and flavor)
1 carrot, cut into large
 chunks
1 turnip, cut into large
 chunks

2 large baking potatoes
5 cups **Vegetable Stock**
2 tablespoons rice vinegar,
 or to taste
1½ cups sour cream
2 tablespoons chopped
 fresh dill

Scrub beets, carrot, turnip and potatoes to remove surface dirt. Place vegetable stock in a large pot, bring to a boil, add beets, carrot and turnip, and boil until they are easily pierced with a fork. Test carrot and turnip after 15 minutes. Remove them from the pot when done. The beets may take half an hour more than the carrot and turnip before they are tender. Continue cooking the beets until done. Total cooking time should be about 1 hour.

Rinse carrot and turnip under cold water and peel. When beets are tender, remove from stock, rinse and peel. Cut beets, carrot and turnip into thin julienne. Return vegetables to stock and add vinegar.

Meanwhile, boil potatoes until fork-tender and cut each into 2 or 4 pieces.

To serve, put borscht into bowls, add 1 or 2 pieces of potato, a dollop of sour cream and a sprinkling of dill.

YIELD: 4 servings

Zuppa di Pomodori con Pesto
(Tomato Soup with Pesto)

2 tablespoons unsalted
   butter
3 onions, diced
3 cloves garlic, minced
1 stalk fennel, diced
3 pounds tomatoes,
   seeded and cubed
4 sprigs parsley

3 sprigs fresh thyme
   (or 2 teaspoons dried)
Freshly ground white
   pepper, to taste
2 cups water or **Vegetable
   Stock**
1 cup heavy cream
1 cup sour cream
³/₄ cup **Basic Basil Pesto**

In a large saucepan, melt butter until foaming. Add onions, garlic and fennel, and cook until wilted (about 15 minutes).

Add tomatoes, parsley, thyme and white pepper, and cook 5 minutes more, stirring gently. Stir in water or stock, bring to a boil and simmer for 30 minutes or until tomatoes are tender. Puree in a food processor or put through a food mill. Reheat; add cream and sour cream. Serve with a dollop of pesto in the center of each serving.

YIELD: 3 to 4 servings

TOMATOES: *Do not peel cooked tomatoes because the peels aid digestion.*

Soupe au Pistou
(Vegetable Soup with Basil Sauce)

Pistou is the French version of pesto and is an equally delicious concoction.

4 to 5 leeks (depending on size)
1 celery root, minced
7 carrots, sliced into thin rounds
2 ounces ($^1/_2$ stick) unsalted butter
3 quarts boiling water

1 cauliflower, cut into florets
$^1/_2$ pound potatoes, washed, boiled, peeled and cut into chunks
Freshly ground white pepper, to taste
$^1/_2$ cup heavy cream (optional)

Pistou:

$^1/_2$ cup fresh basil leaves, tightly packed

3 cloves garlic
Olive oil

Wash vegetables. (Trim leeks to within one inch of the white. Cut leeks in half lengthwise and wash out all the sand.)

Melt butter in a large saucepan. Shake leeks dry, finely mince, and sauté until softened and wilted. Add celery root and carrots. Stir until coated with butter.

Add water, cauliflower and potatoes. Bring to a boil and simmer until all vegetables are tender.

Drain vegetables, reserving stock, and put in food processor or food mill; puree them to a heavy, creamy consistency. Whisk puree into stock.

Make the pistou by placing basil and garlic in a food processor and pulsing for 1 minute. Then with processor running, dribble in oil, using only enough to form a thick paste.

Reheat soup, season with white pepper and whisk in cream at the last minute. Serve Provençal style with a dollop of pistou in the center of each serving.

YIELD: 6 servings

Potage Germiny
(Sorrel Soup)

A soup with the deliciously tart taste of this wild herb.

1 leek
4 tablespoons unsalted
  butter
1 pound sorrel leaves
4 tablespoons flour
*5 cups **Vegetable Stock***

3 egg yolks
³/₄ cup heavy cream
Freshly ground white
  pepper, to taste

Trim leek, leaving about 1 inch of green above the bulb. Cut in half lengthwise and wash in running cold water until free of sand. Shake dry and mince.

In a large soup pot, melt butter until foaming. Add minced leek and sauté until wilted but not brown.

Strip sorrel leaves from stems. Wash and dry leaves, then mince.

Stir sorrel leaves into leeks and cook until wilted. Sprinkle flour over the mixture and stir until combined. Bring stock to a boil. Remove soup pot from heat and slowly pour sorrel mixture in the stock, whisking constantly as you pour so that flour does not lump.

Return soup pot to the stove and, whisking occasionally, simmer soup until heated through and thickened.

Meanwhile, in a medium bowl, beat egg yolks with cream until thickened. Tablespoon by tablespoon, whisk in 1 cup of the soup. Return this egg-soup mixture to the soup pot and whisk it all together over very low heat. (Do not let the soup boil now or the eggs will curdle.) Season with white pepper.

Serve immediately.

YIELD: 4 to 5 servings

Gazpacho

4 to 5 large tomatoes	3 tablespoons rice vinegar
½ cucumber	½ teaspoon freshly ground
½ green bell pepper	black pepper
1 slice onion	⅛ teaspoon cumin
6 tablespoons olive oil	seeds

Using blender or food processor, blend together tomatoes, cucumber, green pepper, onion, oil, vinegar, pepper and cumin seeds until soup consistency is obtained. Chill.*

Serve with diced tomatoes, cucumber and green pepper as condiments.

YIELD: 2 servings

---

* Chilling time will depend on the thickness and quality of the vegetables, and on how well seasoned you like them. The longer gazpacho chills, the stronger the flavor.

Simple Spinach Soup

2 bunches spinach,   3 cloves garlic
  washed and drained   6 sprigs parsley or
1 potato   cilantro
1 carrot   3 cups water
1 slice onion   Cayenne pepper, to taste

Chop vegetables, garlic and parsley by hand or in food processor. Add all ingredients except cayenne to saucepan. Bring to boil; reduce to simmer and cook 10 minutes. Add cayenne and serve.

YIELD: Approximately 4 cups

Red Rice Soup

4 cups **Vegetable Stock**
6 plum tomatoes, diced
1 cup jasmine or basmati
  rice
1 green pepper, diced
3 tablespoons sesame oil
1 large yellow onion, diced
2 cloves garlic, minced

1 tablespoon chili powder
2 teaspoons ground cumin
1 teaspoon ground
  coriander
$^1/_2$ cup coarsely chopped
  cilantro
Sour cream

In a 2 quart sauce pan combine 2 cups stock and diced tomatoes. Bring to boil and add rice and green pepper. Stir to combine. Return to boil and reduce heat. Cover and simmer for 20 minutes.

While rice is cooking, add sesame oil to a large stock pot. When hot add onion, garlic, chili powder, cumin and coriander. Cook over medium heat until onions are transparent and spices are aromatic. Add remaining vegetable stock and cilantro. Bring to a boil then reduce heat and simmer.

Add cooked rice to stock mixture. Stir to combine and simmer gently for 5 minutes to combine flavors. Serve immediately garnished with sour cream.

YIELD: 4 servings

SIX

Soups on the
Protein Side

Stocks

"Make my own stocks? You must be kidding!" That's not an unusual response when I suggest the following recipes to friends and clients. That is, until they have had a chance to taste a homemade stock!

In French, the word for stock, *fonds*, means foundation. And, indeed, a good stock is the base on which many a great meal is built.

Because making stock is time consuming, it is wise to prepare it in large quantities and store it in pint or quart containers in the freezer so it is always at hand when needed.

Fonds de Volaille
(Chicken Stock)

8 quarts cold water
2 4-pound chickens, cut
into pieces, plus the
necks, gizzards, hearts
and feet if possible
(do not include liver)
3 large or 5 small shallots,
cut in quarters
10 cloves
5 garlic cloves, crushed
in the husk

10 peppercorns
10 sprigs fresh thyme
(or 2 tablespoons dried)
1 small bunch fresh dill
(or 2 tablespoons dried)
10 sprigs fresh parsley
(the flat Italian variety
is the most flavorful)
4 bay leaves

Place all ingredients in water, bring to a boil and skim off impurities that rise to the surface.

Lower heat and simmer for 2 hours. Pour through a fine-mesh strainer into a large bowl. Cool uncovered.

Remove all fat from stock and use quart containers to freeze whatever portion of stock is not used immediately.

YIELD: 6 to 7 quarts

Fonds Brun
(Brown Veal Stock)

5 pounds veal bones
4 large or 7 small shallots,
   cut in quarters
10 cloves
1/2 cup minced fresh chives
5 garlic cloves, crushed
   in the husk

10 peppercorns
10 sprigs fresh thyme
   (or 2 tablespoons dried)
10 sprigs fresh parsley
   (the flat Italian variety
   is the most flavorful)
4 bay leaves

Preheat oven to 475°F. Place veal bones in a large roasting pan and brown in preheated oven for 30 minutes. Remove bones to a large stockpot, cover with cold water to about 2 to 3 inches above bones, bring to a boil and skim off impurities that rise to the surface. Lower heat and simmer until water appears clear and nothing rises to the surface.

Add shallots, cloves, chives, garlic, peppercorns, thyme, parsley and bay leaves.

Return stock to a boil. Reduce heat and allow to simmer over very low heat for 24 hours. From time to time, skim fat off top of stock.

Pour finished stock into a large bowl through a fine-mesh strainer. Let stand uncovered until cool, remove any fat that accumulates on the top and return to clean stockpot. Boil and reduce by at least one-third to intensify flavor.

YIELD: Approximately 6 quarts

Demi-Glace

A demi-glace is a reduced stock used to enrich a sauce or pan juices. It is whisked in, the heat is raised and the sauce or pan juices are reduced by boiling at the end of the cooking time.

In a heavy saucepan, place 4 cups of **Fonds de Volaille** or **Fonds Brun**, raise heat to high and boil until stock is reduced by half. You can freeze demi-glace in small containers until needed.

YIELD: Approximately 2 cups

Glace de Volaille or Glace de Viande

This is an even more intense enrichment of a stock, actually made from a demi-glace that is further reduced. Use it to flavor sauces or pan juices by stirring in during final cooking period, raising heat and enriching at the last moment with heavy cream.

In a heavy saucepan, reduce 4 cups of **Demi-Glace** over high heat until all that remains is a heavy, syrupy glaze. Freeze in ice-cube trays. When frozen, place cubes in a plastic bag, where they will always be available to enrich the flavors of sauces used with protein dishes.

YIELD: 1 cup (yield will vary depending on ingredients and desired consistency)

Fumet de Poisson
(Fish Stock)

Fish stock is easy and delicious. It provides a flavorful beginning for many dishes and a delicious addition to many more.

4 pounds fish bones and heads from any fresh white-fleshed fish, such as sole or flounder (it must be a non-oily variety)
6 shallots, quartered
6 sprigs Italian parsley

3 bay leaves
4 sprigs fresh thyme (or 1 tablespoon dried)
10 black peppercorns, lightly crushed
2 tablespoons fennel seeds, crushed

If using fish heads, remove the gills (they can impart a bitter flavor). Several hours ahead or the night before preparing fumet, cover the fish bones with ice water and refrigerate. This will disgorge the blood from the bones.

In a large casserole or stockpot, place the fish bones and heads, the shallots, parsley, bay leaves, thyme, peppercorns and fennel seeds. Add water to cover and slowly bring to a boil. Reduce heat and simmer 20 minutes.

Remove from heat and strain through a fine-mesh sieve.

YIELD: 6 quarts

Court Bouillon

A court bouillon is an aromatic liquid commonly used to poach a whole fish, a fish steak or a fish fillet. Here is my favorite, a variation using clam juice.

6 quarts water
1 cup clam juice (make
    your own by steaming
    clams and reserving
    their cooking broth)
4 shallots, peeled and
    quartered
10 peppercorns
3 garlic cloves, mashed
    flat with the side of a
    chef's knife

5 sprigs Italian parsley
2 bay leaves
4 sprigs thyme
    (or 1 tablespoon dried)
2 tablespoons fennel
    seeds, crushed
1 tablespoon red
    pepper flakes
Freshly ground white
    pepper, to taste

Combine all the ingredients in a fish poacher or a pot large enough to hold the fish to be poached. (A large roasting pan will serve perfectly well.)

Bring to a boil, then reduce heat and barely simmer for 30 minutes, until all the flavors are gently blended.

Allow court bouillon to cool before using it to poach your fish.

YIELD: 6 quarts

Bouillabaisse

This Provençal shellfish-and-seafood stew is fragrant with the essence of garlic.

20 cups fish stock or **Fumet de Poisson**
2 tablespoons fennel seeds, crushed
6 tablespoons chopped garlic
5 sprigs fresh thyme (or 1½ tablespoons dried)
4 sprigs fresh parsley
2 teaspoons paprika
Freshly ground black pepper, to taste
½ teaspoon cayenne pepper
¾ teaspoon saffron threads, crushed

2 large lobsters (1½ to 2 pounds each), cooked, cracked and cut apart at joints
2 pounds each of 3 different kinds of firm, white-fleshed fish of a non-oily variety (tilapia, cod, rockfish, halibut), cut into chunks
1 pound littleneck clams
1 pound mussels
2 pounds sea scallops, cut in quarters, or whole bay scallops

Place stock in a large stockpot. Add fennel, garlic, thyme, parsley, paprika, black pepper, cayenne and saffron; bring to a boil and cook for 30 minutes.

Add lobster pieces and simmer for 5 minutes; add cubed fish and simmer for an additional 5 minutes. Add the clams, mussels and scallops, and cook 5 minutes longer.

Serve bouillabaisse with a bowl of **Sauce Rouille** passed around the table for your guests to enjoy.

YIELD: 4 servings

Clam Soup

4 pounds littleneck clams	1 cup water or **Fumet**
3 sprigs parsley	**de Poisson**
2 cloves garlic, minced	2 egg yolks
2 shallots, minced	1 cup heavy cream
1 bay leaf	½ teaspoon saffron
½ teaspoon red	2 tablespoons minced
pepper flakes	fresh parsley

Scrub clams and soak them in cold water. This encourages clams to open and disgorge their sand. Change the water a few times until all traces of sand disappear.

Place the parsley, garlic, shallots, bay leaf and red pepper flakes in a large saucepan. Add clams and water or stock, cover, and, over medium heat, bring to a boil. Steam clams just until they open. This should take no longer than about 5 minutes. Overcooked clams become tough, so be careful to remove the clams with a skimmer as they open. Shell clams, mince and set aside.

Bring the broth that remains to a boil and reduce by about one-quarter to one-half.

Remove 4 tablespoons of broth from the pot; cool slightly. Beat egg yolks in a small bowl and whisk in the 4 tablespoons of broth to make a liaison or thickener. Set aside.

Add cream and saffron to the clam broth reduction, raise heat, and boil until thickened slightly. Off heat, stir in egg liaison. Distribute minced clams equally among soup bowls and pour soup over. Serve garnished with minced parsley.

YIELD: 4 servings

Mouclades
(Breton Mussel Soup with Cream and Saffron)

4 pounds live mussels	1 cup fish stock or
2 cloves garlic, minced	**Fumet de Poisson**
½ cup shallots, minced	1 cup heavy cream
1 bay leaf	1 egg yolk
3 or 4 sprigs fresh thyme	Pinch of saffron
(or 1 tablespoon dried)	Pinch of ground star
3 or 4 sprigs fresh parsley,	anise (or 2 tablespoons
coarsely chopped	fennel seeds, crushed)
Freshly ground black	
pepper, to taste	

Scrub mussels and remove their "beards," or byssuses, threadlike attachments the mussels use to anchor themselves. Discard any open ones.

In a large heavy saucepan or small stockpot, combine mussels, garlic, shallots, bay leaf, thyme, parsley, pepper and fish stock. Cover with a tight-fitting lid and, over a medium-high flame, steam the mussels until they open. Remove mussels from broth with a skimmer, set aside and keep warm.

Strain mussel broth through a fine sieve, return to saucepan, place over high heat and reduce by about one-quarter. Add heavy cream, raise heat and whisk until broth begins to thicken.

Beat egg yolk. Off heat, remove $1/2$ cup broth to a small bowl and whisk it into the egg yolk by tablespoons. Add saffron and star anise or fennel. Return this mixture to pot of broth and reheat, stirring constantly; do not allow to boil or egg will curdle.

Divide mussels among individual soup bowls, pour soup over them and serve immediately.

YIELD: 4 servings

Soupe de Poisson
(Fish Soup)

1 pound live mussels
*1 1/2 pounds littleneck
  clams*
1/4 cup olive oil
1 cup shallots, minced
*3 tablespoons minced
  garlic*
*1 teaspoon saffron
  threads*
*3 to 4 cups fish stock
  or* **Fumet de Poisson**
1 bay leaf

1 tablespoon fresh thyme
Pinch of cayenne pepper
2 star anise pods
*Freshly ground white
  pepper, to taste*
1 pound skinless fish fillets
1/2 cup heavy cream
*2 tablespoons fennel
  seeds, crushed*
Sauce Rouille

Scrub mussels and remove their beards. Also scrub clams, keeping them separate from the mussels.

Heat oil in a large heavy saucepan or casserole. Add shallots and garlic, and sauté gently until wilted. Rub saffron threads gently between your fingers and add to shallots and garlic.

Add stock, bay leaf, thyme, cayenne, star anise pods and white pepper, and bring to a boil. Simmer for 10 minutes. Add fish fillets and cook 5 minutes longer, keeping water at a gentle simmer.

Place mussels in a medium saucepan with 1/4 cup water and steam until opened (about 5 minutes). Reserve cooking liquid.

Repeat this procedure with clams, again reserving cooking liquid.

Add the mussels, clams and their cooking liquid to soup. Bring to a boil, lower flame, stir in cream and heat through.

Serve in individual soup bowls topped with a sprinkling of crushed fennel seeds. Pass sauce rouille with the soupe de poisson.

YIELD: 4 servings

SEVEN

Pasta with Pleasure

Pasta constitutes the ultimate in eating pleasure! Consider the glorious delights of fettuccine or fettucelle tossed in a white truffle sauce or a delicate herb pasta in a light béchamel, thinned with heavy cream. Try tiny shells (conchigliette) or little bow ties (farfalle) in olive oil and garlic with lightly sautéed crunchy garden vegetables.

To find out just how varied pasta with pleasure can be, don't be shy about trying new and different dishes. A delightful variety of nothing-but-pasta cookbooks abound and are sure to spark your imagination even further than I have and keep your creative, as well as digestive, juices flowing.

Whenever possible, buy fresh pasta, or why not try making it yourself. Visit your nearest supermarket, and you will more than likely find a large selection of fresh and frozen pastas to choose from—everything from the finest capelli d'angelo (angel hair) to a hearty dark-green spinach lasagna.

When using dry pasta, higher quality generally means much better taste and texture. Health food stores have whole-wheat and artichoke flour pastas, which are fine. My personal favorite brand, which is carried in almost all grocery stores, is De Cicco, made with semolina and imported from Italy. Do not buy pasta made with soy flour, salt or eggs.

If the pasta is fresh, leave it at room temperature, uncovered, for up to one day or freeze it. Some groceries sell refrigerated pasta; they will advise you on how long it can be kept. A pound of fresh pasta will typically yield about 6 cups after cooking.

Cook according to package directions, though I suggest using about 6 quarts of water for every pound of pasta. Ordinarily, dried pasta will increase in bulk by about half when cooked. Add a dash of oil to the boiling water and cook until pasta reaches the *al dente* ("to the tooth") stage—until still slightly firm. To test for doneness, remove a piece of pasta from the water, cool and then bite into it. If the pasta is cooked through but still offers a slight resistance to the tooth, it's done—drain and serve immediately. Cooking time will vary with the thickness of the particular pasta. Usually it takes about 8 to 10 minutes.

Drain and toss with desired sauce. I prefer not to rinse pasta with cold water unless I am baking the dish later or letting it cool. Some people, however, prefer to rinse it.

Fettuccine with White Truffles

ᦔ

1 ounce white truffles
1 tablespoon olive oil
1 pound fettuccine
1 cup cold water

5 tablespoons unsalted
  butter
Freshly ground white
  pepper, to taste

Slice truffles paper-thin and reserve any juice. (It is best to use a special truffle slicer for this purpose; the slicer enables you to shave them paper-thin for the fullest taste.)

In a large pot of boiling water to which you have added oil, add fettuccine and cook, stirring occasionally, just until pasta is al dente. (If fettuccine is fresh, this will be less than 1 minute after pasta is added and water returns to a boil. Dried fettuccine will take about 8 to 10 minutes at a full rolling boil.)

Immediately add 1 cup cold water to boiling pasta to stop the cooking. Drain.

In a large sauté pan, melt butter. Add drained pasta and toss. Top with white pepper, truffles and any reserved truffle juice.

Serve immediately.

YIELD: 4 servings

TRUFFLES: *I said you can have it all—and that really should include truffles. If you haven't tasted these unforgettable treats, you really should. You deserve it!*

Truffles are brown, roundish fruiting bodies. Along with mushrooms, they belong to the family of plants known as fungi. The primary difference is that mushrooms grow on the surface of the ground, while truffles grow underground—making them difficult to find and very expensive.

The aroma and taste of truffles is so intense—and their cost so great—that they are best used sparingly as a flavoring instead of a separate dish.

White truffles should be eaten raw, cut in very fine slices and served as a topping on preparations that have already been cooked. Truffles should be held for no more than a few days before consuming. Store them loosely wrapped in paper towels or in a closed jar filled with raw rice (which can later be used to make a delicious risotto).

Trenette con Funghi
(Narrow Noodles with Wild Mushrooms)

4 tablespoons unsalted butter	1 teaspoon fresh rosemary (or ½ teaspoon dried)
5 tablespoons olive oil	1½ ounces dried wild mushrooms (porcini, morels, chanterelles or a combination)
¼ cup minced onion	
2 tablespoons minced shallot	
3 cloves garlic, minced	Freshly ground white pepper, to taste
¼ cup tomato paste	½ cup heavy cream
2 to 3 cups **Vegetable Stock**	1 pound trenette (narrow, flat ribbon noodles)
3 bay leaves	

Heat butter and oil in a sauté pan until melted. Add onion, shallot and garlic, and sauté until lightly colored. Add tomato paste; whisk together.

Add 2 cups stock, bay leaves and rosemary. Simmer on low flame until thickened, about 45 minutes to 1 hour. (Add more stock to thin sauce, if necessary.)

Meanwhile, soak dried mushrooms in 1 cup water for about ½ hour. Drain and dry. Cut into bite-size chunks.

Start heating large pot of water. While waiting for it to boil, stir mushrooms into sauce. Add white pepper and cream. Cook trenette until just al dente. (If trenette is fresh, start testing for doneness about 5 seconds after water returns to a boil.) Meanwhile, heat sauce just to boiling.

Drain trenette, add sauce and serve.
YIELD: 4 servings

EASY PEELING: *To peel a garlic clove, gently flatten it by hand or with the flat side of a chef's knife; the peel will then release easily. Cut off the end and discard any green parts— they tend to be bitter. Browning also makes garlic somewhat bitter, but I'm among those people who like it that way.*

Pasta Rosa alla Panna
(Red Pasta in Butter and Cream Sauce)

Try to find pasta rosa for this recipe. It's a fresh pasta made with pureed beets, giving it a luscious deep red color that's lovely to see when tossed with the delicate white cream sauce.

1 tablespoon olive oil	8 tablespoons unsalted
1 pound pasta rosa	butter (approximately)
(spinach fettuccine may	4 egg yolks
be substituted)	½ cup heavy cream

Bring a large pot of water to a boil. Add oil and cook pasta until just al dente.

While pasta is boiling, melt 2 tablespoons butter in a sauté pan.

In a small bowl, whisk the yolks together until thickened. Then whisk in heavy cream and set aside.

When pasta is ready, drain thoroughly. Run under cool water, drain again and add it to the sauté pan. Add 4 to 6 more tablespoons butter and toss. Pour on the egg-yolk-and-cream sauce and toss very quickly. Heat through but do not allow to cook or the egg will curdle.

Serve immediately.

YIELD: 4 servings

Aglio e Olio
(Pasta with Garlic and Olive Oil)

1 pound spaghetti,	*2 to 3 large cloves garlic,*
fettuccine or linguine	*peeled and minced*
½ cup olive oil, plus oil	*Freshly ground black*
for cooking water	*pepper, to taste*

Cook pasta in several quarts boiling water with a few drops of oil. Cook to al dente stage and drain thoroughly.

Heat oil and toss in cooked pasta. Cook 1 to 2 minutes over medium-low heat. Toss in garlic* and cook 30 seconds over low heat. Add a few grindings of fresh pepper.

YIELD: 2 servings

---

* Some cooks recommend sautéing the garlic in oil first; if you do sauté it, use caution and don't brown it, or it will be bitter. Cook only until slightly golden, then add to pasta.

Pasta with Butter and Garlic

1 pound spaghetti,
   fettuccine or linguine
1 teaspoon olive oil
½ cup (1 stick) unsalted
   butter

2 to 3 large cloves garlic,
   minced
Freshly ground black
   pepper, to taste

Cook pasta in several quarts boiling water with the oil. Cook to al dente stage and drain thoroughly.

Heat butter in a large skillet but do not brown it. Toss in pasta and cook 1 to 2 minutes on low heat, or just until pasta is hot. Toss in garlic and cook 30 seconds. Add pepper and serve.

YIELD: 2 servings

Pasta with Sautéed Vegetables

8 large mushrooms,
   cleaned and sliced
½ cup plus 2 tablespoons
   olive oil
10 broccoli florets,
   blanched 2 minutes
   and refreshed*
10 asparagus spears, cut
   diagonally, blanched 2
   minutes and refreshed*

1 pound spaghetti, cooked
   and drained**
2 large cloves garlic,
   minced
Freshly ground black
   pepper, to taste

Sauté mushrooms in 1 tablespoon hot oil for 1 to 2 minutes; set aside. Sauté broccoli 1 minute in 1½ teaspoons hot oil. Sauté asparagus 1 minute in 1½ teaspoons hot oil.

Heat ½ cup oil. Sauté pasta 1 to 2 minutes. Add vegetables and garlic, and cook 1 minute. Add pepper and serve.

YIELD: 2 servings

---

* "To refresh" means to rinse under cold water.

** Some people cook the pasta in the water in which they have blanched the vegetables.

Pasta with Peas

1 cup finely chopped
   onion
¹/₄ cup butter
¹/₄ cup olive oil
2 cloves garlic, finely
   chopped
10 ounces small pasta
   shells, cooked and
   drained

2 ¹/₂ cups cooked peas
1 cup finely chopped
   fresh parsley
Freshly ground black
   pepper, to taste

Sauté onion in butter and oil for 6 to 8 minutes. Add garlic and cook very slowly for another moment or two. Remove from heat, add pasta, peas, parsley and pepper. Mix well to serve.

YIELD: 2 servings

Lasagna

*1 pound lasagna noodles,
cooked, drained and
rinsed in cold water
1 to 2 yellow onions,
chopped and sautéed in
2 tablespoons butter*

*30 mushrooms, sliced and
sautéed in 3 to 5 table-
spoons butter
1 recipe **Pesto for Pasta**
at room temperature*

Layer noodles, onions and mushrooms in baking dish (you will probably want 3 layers of pasta and 2 layers of vegetables). Drizzle layers with a bit of pesto. Bake uncovered for 25 minutes at 350°F. Spoon on remaining pesto to serve.*

YIELD: 2 servings

Variation 1: Super Veggie Lasagna

If you prefer more vegetables in proportion to the pasta, try adding sautéed zucchini, broccoli or spinach to the mushroom layers.

Variation 2: Onion Lasagna

If you wish, substitute 1 recipe **Mazel "Cheese" Italian** for the chopped onions. You will then have more onions in the lasagna.

---

* Vegetable lasagna is delicious, nutritious and a boon if you are entertaining because you can refrigerate it after preparing and then bake it whenever you are ready to serve.

Gnocchi with Sage Butter

Sage Butter:

½ cup unsalted butter	2 cloves garlic, minced
4 tablespoons finely chopped fresh sage leaves (or 2 tablespoons dried)	

Melt butter; add sage and garlic. Cook over gentle heat for 5 minutes. Let butter stand for about 1 hour to develop flavor.

Gnocchi:

1½ pounds boiling potatoes, unpeeled	1½ cups flour
	½ tablespoon oil

Boil potatoes until tender when pierced with a fork; drain and peel. Puree in a food processor or put through ricer while still warm.

Place pureed potatoes in a bowl and slowly add flour until mixture is smooth and homogeneous but still sticky.

Shape dough by rolling into long, narrow sausage-like shapes about the diameter of a nickel. Keep work area lightly floured. Then, with a sharp knife, cut diagonally into pieces about 1-inch long.

Bend into small crescent shapes.

Add gnocchi to 5 quarts of rapidly boiling water to which you have added oil to prevent sticking; stir.

When gnocchi rise to surface, allow to cook 1 more minute, then remove with slotted spoon and drain.

Serve gnocchi with warm sage butter poured over them.

YIELD: 4 servings

Variation:

You will also enjoy gnocchi served with a marinara sauce.

Risotto alla Milanese
(Rice in the Style of Milan)

In a perfectly cooked risotto, each grain of rice is creamy but still distinct and al dente—a balance of qualities best achieved with Arborio, a particularly plump, pearly, short-grained rice from Italy. Capable of absorbing an uncommonly large amount of cooking liquid while still retaining a nugget of resistance, Arborio is the rice of choice for this famous dish.

3 tablespoons unsalted butter, softened	Pinch of oregano
1 tablespoon minced onion	Pinch of thyme
	Freshly ground white pepper, to taste
1 clove garlic, minced	Pinch of saffron threads
1 cup Arborio rice	½ cup heavy cream,
4 cups water or **Vegetable Stock**	room temperature

In a covered, 4- to 6-quart heavy pot, melt 2 tablespoons of the butter until bubbling gently. Add onion and garlic, and sauté over low heat until onion is softened.

Stir in rice, coating completely with butter and onion; continue stirring for several minutes. Then add 1 cup of the water or stock, mixing well and stirring until the liquid is absorbed.

Stir in oregano, thyme and pepper. Rub the saffron threads between your thumb and forefinger, and dissolve in 1 cup of stock. Add stock with saffron to rice and stir gently until all moisture is absorbed.

Continue adding stock, stirring constantly, and cook until rice is tender but still chewy. (It may not be necessary to use all liquid called for in the list of ingredients.)

Fold in remaining tablespoon softened butter and heavy cream. Serve immediately.

YIELD: 4 servings

Risotto con Asparagi
(Rice with Asparagus)

*1 pound fresh young
asparagus, washed
and lightly peeled**
*3 tablespoons unsalted
butter*
*1 tablespoon minced
onion or shallot*
1 clove garlic, minced
*1 cup Arborio rice (see
Risotto alla Milanese)*

*Freshly ground black pepper,
to taste*
*4 cups water or **Vegetable
Stock***
1 cup heavy cream
*2 tablespoons fresh
savory or thyme
(or 1 tablespoon dried)*

Slice asparagus into ½-inch lengths diagonally.

Make risotto as described in recipe for Risotto alla Milanese, but add the sliced asparagus to the sauté of onion, garlic and rice. If using dried herbs, add at this time.

When the risotto is ready, fold in fresh herbs and serve.

YIELD: 4 servings

---

* Almost any vegetable can be substituted for the asparagus.

EIGHT

Pastry with Permission

Pâte Feuilletée Fine
(Puff Pastry)

4 ½ cups unbleached
   flour (use dry measur-
   ing cups, dipped and
   leveled)
1 ⅓ cups water
10 ½ tablespoons
   unsalted butter, melted

1 pound (4 sticks)
   unsalted butter
Additional flour for
   kneading surface

Place 2 to 3 cups of the flour in a large bowl and form a well in the center. Add water and melted butter to the well. Starting at the center of the well, use your fingers to mix flour into liquid center, beginning with a small amount and gradually adding more and more flour to the liquid, until you have used all 4½ cups of flour. Form this mass into a ball; knead once or twice. Form into a 1½-inch-high square, wrap in plastic wrap and refrigerate for 30 minutes.

Lightly flour 1 pound butter. Place lengthwise between two sheets of wax paper and begin flattening and elongating the butter by tapping it with a heavy rolling pin. When butter is approximately 5 x 12 inches, fold it in three by scraping it up and turning it over onto itself as you would a business letter. Make a quarter turn of the butter and repeat the procedure: Flour the surface on both top and bottom, place between two sheets of wax paper and begin tapping it out to elongate.

The butter must remain cold, or it will begin to stick to the paper and will take too much flour to roll and elongate. So work quickly and press it out as evenly as possible, repeating this procedure 4 or 5 times until butter is an elongated rectangle of approximately 5 x 12 inches. Refrigerate for 15 minutes.

It is essential that both the flour mixture and the butter be at approximately the same temperature because they will now be folded together and the butter must not under any circumstances bleed through the flour mixture.

On a pastry marble (which will maintain the cold temperature of the pastry for the longest period of time), roll out the flour mixture to a size approximately 4 inches longer and wider than the butter. This will allow enough room to enclose the butter when it is laid over the flour mixture. Place the rectangle of butter in the center of the flour mixture, fold the edges up over the butter so they meet and press the pastry together to seal the butter inside. Now, with a heavy rolling pin, roll the pastry into a somewhat larger rectangle, approximately 20 inches long. From the bottom up, fold the pastry into thirds as you would a business letter; give the pastry a quarter-turn clockwise and repeat the rolling/folding procedure. You have now given the pastry two turns. Wrap in plastic wrap and refrigerate to rest the dough and relax the gluten in the flour so that the dough will not shrink back when rolled.

After a rest of about 1 hour, place the pastry on the floured work surface and repeat the rolling and folding procedure for two more turns. Refrigerate, wrapped in plastic wrap, for 2 hours.

Make two more turns, so that you've completed six in all. The pastry is now ready to use. Keep it chilled until ready to roll it.

YIELD: Approximately 6 to 8 entrée-size servings

Puff Pastry Tourte with Leek and Mushroom Filling

2 pounds leeks	Freshly ground or grated
6 tablespoons unsalted	nutmeg
butter	³/₄ pound mushrooms,
1½ tablespoons flour	sliced
³/₄ cup heavy cream	1 recipe **Pâte Feuilletée**
Freshly ground white	**Fine** (keep pastry cold
pepper, to taste	until ready to roll and fill)
Pinch of cayenne pepper	1 egg yolk beaten with
2 teaspoons fresh thyme	1 tablespoon water
(or 1 teaspoon dried)	

Preheat oven to 475°F.

To prepare the filling, make two long, crosswise slices down through the green of the leeks and a little way into the white. Wash carefully under cold running water to make sure you've removed all the sand. Slice the leeks into very thin rounds. Melt 2 tablespoons butter in a heavy sauté pan and cook leeks over moderate heat, stirring occasionally, until they begin to wilt but not brown. Add 2 more tablespoons butter, cover and slowly steam leeks in butter. Uncover, stir in flour; blend well. Cook for 3 or 4 more minutes and set aside.

Place cream in a small heavy saucepan and cook over high heat until reduced by half. Stir the cream into leeks and add white pepper, cayenne, thyme and nutmeg. Reheat, stirring until thickened.

Melt remaining 2 tablespoons butter in a sauté pan and add mushrooms. Sauté until mushrooms are lightly browned and all moisture has evaporated. Stir into leek mixture and set aside.

You will need only two-thirds of the puff pastry for this recipe. Cut in three; reserve two sections and freeze the third. On a floured marble or pastry board, roll out one piece of pastry until it is ⅛-inch thick. This is the bottom. Using a 9-inch vol-au-vent round pastry cutter or a 9-inch pot cover, cut out a circle of pastry. Place circle on a buttered cookie sheet that has been sprinkled with cold water. Place leek and mushroom mixture in a mound in the center of the pastry. With a pastry brush and water, paint a circle around the mound of filling, taking care not to allow it to drip over the edge of the dough circle. (This would cause the layers of dough to stick together and inhibit the rising of the pastry.) Roll out second piece, top half (the cover), of the tourte ¹⁄₁₆ inch thicker than the bottom. Cut as you did the bottom and place over bottom layer and filling, gently pressing all around the outside of the circle of filling to join the two circles of pastry. Poke a steam hole in the top of tourte.

Using the dull side of a small paring knife, scallop the outside edge of the tourte by pressing in the edges of the pastry at 1½-inch intervals. Decorate the top with the sharp side of the knife—without cutting through the pastry, draw curving lines from the center to the outside edge.

With egg-yolk-and-water mixture (the glaze), paint

the top of tourte, taking care not to allow mixture to drip over the edges of tourte.

Bake at 475°F for 20 minutes, then reduce temperature to 400°F and bake for 35 minutes longer or until golden brown and cooked through. If you think the top or part of the top is browning too quickly toward the end of the cooking time, cover that part loosely with aluminum foil.

Serve immediately.

YIELD: 6 to 8 servings

Variation: Spinach-Dill Tourte

Substitute 2 pounds chopped spinach and 2 tablespoons chopped fresh dill for the leeks.

Feuilletées
(Individual Puff Pastry Shells)

Individual feuilletées can be prepared in advance, frozen raw and then simply popped into the oven and baked just before serving.

1 recipe **Pâte Feuilletée Fine**	1 egg yolk beaten with 1 tablespoon water
1 tablespoon water	

Preheat oven to 475°F.

It is easiest to work with and cut the feuilletées if the puff pastry is divided in three before rolling. Using a large, sharp, floured knife, cut the pastry crosswise into three equal pieces. Refrigerate two of them while working on the other. Flour the work surface and roll out the pastry into a square approximately ⅛-inch thick. Using a ruler, cut pastry into 5-inch squares. Cut off ½-inch strips all around and place the squares on a pastry sheet rinsed with cold water.

Brush the top outside edges of squares with water, taking care not to let water run over the sides of the pastry shell or it will not rise properly. Gently place strips all around edges of pastry squares, overlapping at the corners, and press down lightly. (You are creating a little box which, when it rises, will serve to encase any vegetable filling.) With the blunt side of a small paring knife, lightly press a ¼-inch scallop pattern around the outside edge of the pastry shell. Glaze the borders of this box with egg-water mixture, again being careful not to let the liquid run over the sides. Prick the center of the box with a fork so that it will not rise as high as the outside.

Bake at 475°F for 5 minutes, then reduce temperature to 400°F and bake 8 to 10 minutes longer. Remove to a rack and cool. Carefully scoop out center of square to make room for filling.

Fill with any vegetable puree or any fresh-cooked vegetables in sauce (for example, fresh asparagus tips with hollandaise sauce).

For feuilletées with spinach and dill, simply make the filling for **Spinach-Dill Tourte**, pile into the feuilletées and serve piping hot.

YIELD: 6 servings

Duxelles
(Mushroom Stuffing)

Use duxelles to fill mushroom caps or a puff pastry casing, or simply as a delicious vegetable dish all by itself.

*4 tablespoons unsalted
    butter
1 onion, minced
2 shallots, minced
1 pound mushrooms,
    minced (including stems)*

*Freshly ground black
    pepper, to taste
1 teaspoon fresh thyme,
    oregano or tarragon
    (optional)*

In a medium sauté pan, melt butter over medium heat. Add onion and shallots; sauté gently until wilted. Do not brown.

Add mushrooms and cook over high heat to evaporate all moisture. As they are cooking, shake the pan back and forth over the burner so that the mixture does not stick and the heat is evenly distributed. When moisture has evaporated, the dish is ready to serve.

Season with pepper and fresh herbs, if desired.

YIELD: Approximately 1 cup

Pâte Brisée

This pastry is great for vegetable tarts or tart shells for vegetable purees.

1¼ cups unbleached flour
½ cup whole-wheat pastry flour or unbleached stone-ground pastry flour (available in health food stores)

12 tablespoons (1½ sticks) unsalted butter, frozen
¼ to ⅓ cup ice water*

Combine flours in a food processor and blend for 2 or 3 seconds.

Cut the frozen butter into 12 equal parts and place in the processor.

Pulse 10 or 12 times, or until butter is combined with flour and is broken up into small pea-size pieces. Do not overprocess or pastry will be tough.

With the machine running, add ice water, being sure to add only as much as is needed to make the dough stick together. It will start to gather into a ball on top of the blade.

Remove dough as soon as it forms a ball and stretch out on the work surface to give a final blending to the flour and butter. Shape into a ball and

---

* Flour, even the same brand, will react differently every time you use it. Its moisture content varies considerably, and that, plus weather conditions, which also affect how much liquid it can absorb, will determine how much water you use.

refrigerate for at least 1 hour before rolling. This will give the gluten in the flour the opportunity to relax before rolling.

(This dough can be made in a large bowl if you prefer. Combine the flour, make a well in the center and add cold [but not frozen butter]. Using your fingertips, two knives or a pastry blender, blend with flour until small morsels are formed. Add water, mix and form into a ball. Refrigerate.)

Preheat oven to 450°F.

Generously butter a 9-inch tart tin with removable bottom. (A 9-inch pie tin is also acceptable.) On a floured work surface—a pastry marble is best, but a board will do—roll the dough into a circle approximately 11 to 12 inches in diameter. Roll the dough back onto the rolling pin and unroll gently onto the tart tin. Carefully ease the dough into the tin, pressing into the grooves with your thumb. Move the rolling pin over the top to remove the excess dough. Refrigerate until set, or freeze for 5 minutes. Place a piece of buttered aluminum foil over the dough and gently mold it into the shell. Fill with metal baking beans (if unavailable, rice or dried beans will do) and bake at 450°F for 13 to 14 minutes. Remove foil and beans, and bake for 3 minutes more. You now have a partially baked—or "baked blind"—tart shell, which can be used for any vegetable filling.

YIELD: 1 9-inch or 10-inch tart shell

Champignons Sauvages aux Herbes à la Crème
(Wild Mushrooms with Herbs and Cream)

There are many varieties of wild mushrooms available. If you are unable to find them at a local gourmet shop, many food catalogs and mail-order houses offer them. Watch for advertisements in the backs of home and food magazines, too.

*Puff pastry (**Pâte Feuilletée Fine**) scraps*
1 egg yolk beaten with 1 tablespoon water
1 pound fresh wild mushrooms; choose one variety or combine cèpes, morels, chanterelles and porcini (or 3 to 4 ounces dried)
4 tablespoons unsalted butter
4 tablespoons minced shallot

1 clove garlic, minced
2 tablespoons tarragon (or 1 teaspoon dried)
2 tablespoons thyme (or 1 teaspoon dried)
2 tablespoons chervil (or 1 teaspoon dried)
2 tablespoons fresh Italian parsley
Freshly ground black pepper, to taste
6 tablespoons heavy cream

First, make fleurons—small crescents, about 3 inches in length—from puff pastry scraps (keep pastry scraps in the freezer—never discard them!). Roll out dough, cut out crescents, one for each serving with a cookie or pastry cutter. Paint crescents with glaze of egg yolk and water, place on cookie sheet and bake at

475°F for 5 minutes. Lower heat to 400°F and bake 8 to 10 minutes longer or until puffed and golden.

If mushrooms are dried, soak until softened, drain and wipe dry. This will approximately double their size.

Cut mushrooms into quarters or large bite-size chunks.

Melt butter in a large sauté pan. Add shallot and cook until wilted. Add garlic and sauté briefly.

Place mushrooms in the sauté pan and cook just until heated through (2 or 3 minutes). If exposed to too much heat, they will begin to wilt and lose their moisture.

Sprinkle on the herbs and pepper, and add cream. Toss until well combined, remove from heat and serve immediately on fleurons.

YIELD: 4 servings

Tarte Provençale

2 pounds tomatoes
  (preferably Italian plum
  variety)
4 tablespoons olive oil
4 medium or 5 small
  zucchini
Freshly ground black
  pepper, to taste
2 to 3 cloves garlic
  (to taste), minced

½ cup fresh bread
  crumbs
2 tablespoons chopped
  Italian parsley
1 8- or 9-inch **Pâte Brisée**
  tart shell, baked for
  15 minutes or until set
5 fresh basil leaves,
  minced

Preheat oven to 400°F.

Plunge tomatoes in boiling water for 10 seconds. Peel, slice, seed and dice.

Sauté tomatoes in 1 tablespoon olive oil until just softened and still a bit firm. Remove from pan and set aside.

Cut zucchini into about the same size dice as tomatoes and sauté in 1 tablespoon olive oil until tender but still crunchy. Set alongside tomatoes and grind pepper over both.

Sauté half the garlic in 1 tablespoon olive oil until softened. Add bread crumbs and parsley, and sauté just until fully moistened.

In precooked pastry shell, assemble cooked zucchini and tomatoes; top with basil, remaining minced and sautéed breadcrumb mixture. Dribble remaining

1 tablespoon olive oil over all and bake at 400°F for 20 minutes. Serve immediately.

YIELD: 6 to 7 servings

NINE

Potatoes—
Any Style

Baked, French fries, cottage fries—of course you can have it all! These year-round favorites are at their freshest in the early fall. Your best bet for baking and French fries are russets, while new potatoes are your best pick for boiling and using in salads.

Hot Potato

Bake, split open and season potato with lots of grated fresh horseradish and cayenne.

Baldwin Skins

Bake potatoes, scrape out insides (use for something else) and rub skins with butter. Sprinkle with cayenne and black pepper, and crisp lightly under broiler.

American Potato Salad

Boil, peel and dice potatoes. Dress with chopped scallions, chopped celery, chopped red bell peppers and onions that have been sautéed in oil and cooled. Toss with **Carb Mayonnaise** (made with egg yolk only) to serve.

Italian Potato Salad

Boil, peel and dice potatoes. Sauté chopped red and green bell peppers in olive oil. Toss potatoes and peppers with additional olive oil, crushed fennel seeds and finely chopped garlic. Serve warm. Add pepper and chopped herbs, if desired.

Pesto Potatoes

Use pesto on baked or boiled potatoes.

Potato Latkes 1

4 large unpeeled potatoes
1 onion, peeled
1 tablespoon unsalted
   matzo meal

Freshly ground black
   pepper, to taste
$^1/_2$ to $^1/_4$ cup sesame oil

Rinse potatoes and onion, but do not soak. Grate them finely and squeeze out liquid. Add matzo meal and pepper; toss gently to combine. Allow to sit 1 to 2 minutes so that meal is well moistened. Form into pancakes.

Fry pancakes in small amount of hot oil, pressing them now and then with a spatula until brown and crunchy on both sides. Depending on size, latkes will have to cook about 4 to 5 minutes on each side.

YIELD: 2 servings

Potato Latkes 2

1 small yellow onion,
   peeled
3 large russet potatoes,
   unpeeled

2 tablespoons potato
   flour
Unsalted butter
Sour cream (optional)

Grate onion and potato. Add flour and form into pancakes. Fry in butter. Top with sour cream and serve.

YIELD: 2 servings

Variation: Cinnamon Latkes

Omit the onion and use sour cream and cinnamon as a topping.

Sweet-Potato Fry

2 sweet potatoes or yams
4 carrots, scrubbed
2 leeks, thoroughly
  cleaned
2 tablespoons sesame
  oil

Cinnamon, to taste
Nutmeg, to taste
2 bunches spinach,
  thoroughly cleaned

Cut sweet potatoes into thin, diagonal slices. Cut carrots a bit thicker, also diagonally. Cut leeks diagonally, using the white part and a bit of the tender green part.

In hot oil, stir-fry the potatoes, carrots and leeks until brown and crunchy. Cover and cook over low heat until they are just tender (10 to 15 minutes). Season with cinnamon and nutmeg.

Cook uncovered until crisp again.

Toss in spinach leaves and cook, uncovered, until they wilt (not more than a few seconds).

YIELD: 2 servings

Variation: Buttered Sweet-Potato Fry

Use unsalted butter instead of the safflower oil.

Mazel Potato Salad

3 pounds small new
  potatoes (red-skinned
  make the prettiest
  salad)
1/4 teaspoon dry mustard
Freshly ground white
  pepper, to taste
2 tablespoons rice
  vinegar
1/4 to 1/3 cup oil
  (olive oil, or light-colored
  sesame oil and olive
  oil mixed)

2 tablespoons minced
  fresh tarragon
  (or 1 1/2 teaspoons dried)
1/2 cup minced shallot
1 tablespoon minced
  chervil (or 1 1/2
  teaspoons dried)
3 cloves garlic, minced
2 tablespoons minced
  Italian parsley

Wash potatoes and place in a large saucepan; cover with cold water. Bring to a boil and simmer until just fork-tender (15 to 20 minutes at the most). Drain and let cool just a bit.

While potatoes are boiling, make vinaigrette: Combine mustard, pepper and vinegar. Then whisk in oil until dressing thickens. Add tarragon, shallot, chervil and garlic.

Place vinaigrette in a large bowl and top with the potatoes. Toss. Sprinkle with parsley and serve warm.

YIELD: 4 servings

READER/CUSTOMER CARE SURVEY

If you are enjoying this book, please help us serve you better and meet your changing needs by taking a few minutes to complete this survey. Please fold it & drop it in the mail.

Name: _____

Address: _____

_____

Tel. # _____

As a special **"Thank You"** we'll send you exciting news about interesting books and a valuable Gift Cerficate.
It's Our Pleasure to Serve You!

(1) Gender: 1) ____ Female 2) ____ Male

(2) Age:
1)____ 18-25 4)____ 46-55
2)____ 26-35 5)____ 56-65
3)____ 36-45 6)____ 65+

(3) Marital status:

1)____ Married 3)____ Single 5)____ Widowed
2)____ Divorced 4)____ Partner

(4) Is this book:
1)____ Purchased for self?
2)____ Purchased for others?
3)____ Received as gift?

(5) How did you find out about this book?

1)____ Catalog   2)____ Store Display
Newspaper
3)____ Best Seller List
4)____ Article/Book Review
5)____ Advertisement
Magazine
6)____ Feature Article
7)____ Book Review
8)____ Advertisement
9)____ Word of Mouth
A)____ T.V./Talk Show (Specify) _____
B)____ Radio/Talk Show (Specify) _____
C)____ Professional Referral _____
D)____ Other (Specify) _____

Which Health Communications book are you currently reading? _____

(6) What subject areas do you enjoy reading most? (Rank in order of enjoyment)

1)____ Women's Issues/   5)____ New Age/
        Relationships   Altern. Healing
2)____ Business Self Help   6)____ Aging
3)____ Soul/Spirituality/   7)____ Parenting
        Inspiration   8)____ Diet/Nutrition/
4)____ Recovery   Exercise/Health

(14) What do you look for when choosing a personal growth book?
(Rank in order of importance)
1)____ Subject   3)____ Author
2)____ Title   4)____ Price
       Cover Design   5)____ In Store Location

(19) When do you buy books?
(Rank in order of importance)
1)____ Christmas
2)____ Valentine's Day
3)____ Birthday
4)____ Mother's Day
5)____ Other (Specify _____

(23) Where do you buy your books?
(Rank in order of frequency of purchases)
1)____ Bookstore   6)____ Gift Store
2)____ Price Club   7)____ Book Club
3)____ Department Store 8)____ Mail Order
4)____ Supermarket/   9)____ T.V. Shopping
       Drug Store   A)____ Airport
5)____ Health Food Store

Additional comments you would like to make to help us serve you better.

_____

_____

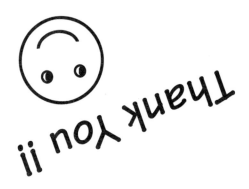

Thank You !!

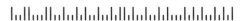

TEN

Open-Carb Combos

Couscous Mazel

8 dried shiitake mushrooms
1 large onion, finely
    chopped
1 bay leaf
2 tablespoons light-
    colored sesame oil
3 garlic cloves, finely
    chopped

1 teaspoon cumin powder
¼ teaspoon dried dill weed
Pinch of cayenne pepper
1 cup cooked couscous
    (see cooking directions
    below)

Soak mushrooms in warm water until soft (about 15 minutes). Squeeze out water and discard hard stems. Cut mushrooms into small pieces.

Sauté onion with bay leaf in oil until soft. Add garlic, mushrooms and spices; sauté until onions are lightly browned.

Mix all ingredients with cooked couscous. Remove bay leaves before serving.

To cook couscous:

1 tablespoon light-colored
    sesame oil
1 bay leaf

1 cup couscous
2½ cups water

Heat oil in sauté pan. Add bay leaf and couscous. Brown lightly, being careful not to burn.

Transfer to a pot with water. Boil until water makes little volcanic gurgles. Lower heat to its minimum, cover pot and cook until water is absorbed (15 to 20 minutes).

YIELD: 2 servings

SHIITAKE MUSHROOMS: *Unlike fresh mushrooms, dried shiitake mushrooms must be soaked in water for 20 to 30 minutes. Use warm water only—hot water tends to make them bitter. Be sure to discard the tough stems.*

Mazel Pizza

Dough:

1 package active dry yeast (or 1 cake compressed fresh yeast)	4 tablespoons olive oil plus 2 teaspoons
1 cup warm water	1 tablespoon crushed fennel seeds
1½ cups unbleached flour	1 teaspoon crushed red pepper flakes
1½ cups whole-wheat flour	

Crumble yeast into water and stir.

Place flours in mixer or food processor (entire dough can also be made by hand); add yeast mixture and 4 tablespoons oil. Mix until dough is soft but not sticky. If necessary, add a bit more flour or a bit more water to attain the proper consistency.

Add fennel and red pepper flakes, then knead dough until smooth and elastic.

Put 2 teaspoons of oil into a clean bowl, add dough and flip to grease all over. Cover bowl with plastic wrap and place in a warm place (about 80°F) to rise until doubled (about 1 to 1½ hours).

Filling and baking:

7 large onions, thinly
  sliced, with slices
  separated
2½ cups good olive oil
2 red bell peppers, sliced
1 green bell pepper, sliced
20 fresh mushrooms,
  coarsely sliced
9 to 10 large garlic cloves,
  peeled and minced
14 Italian plum tomatoes,
  peeled, seeded and
  juiced, coarsely sliced

1 cup extremely thick
  Mazel Marinara*
1 tablespoon crushed
  fennel seeds**
3 tablespoons mixed fresh
  herbs (or 2 teaspoons
  dried), such as parsley,
  thyme, chives and
  oregano
1 tablespoon crushed red
  pepper flakes

Preheat oven to 500°F.

Over low heat, sauté onions in 1½ cups oil for 40 minutes or until very soft; set aside.

Divide dough into three parts for baking in three separate pans (9-inch omelet-shaped pans are perfect; however, if you have only one small oven, you will need pans without handles). Place 3 tablespoons of oil into each pan. On a floured surface, roll out each piece of dough into a thin circle. Roll edges, pressing them to make the outer edges thicker than the bottom of the dough circle. The bottom should be thin.

Sauté red and green bell peppers in 3 tablespoons hot oil for 2 minutes. Remove from pan and set aside. Add 3 tablespoons more oil and sauté mushrooms in

---

* If necessary, reduce your marinara sauce over medium heat until it thickens.
** Herbs and seeds can be crushed with mortar and pestle or with a heavy skillet or wine bottle on a wooden board.

this oil for 1 to 2 minutes on high heat so that they will color. Remove mushrooms and set aside. Turn off heat under oil and add garlic and tomatoes; toss about 30 seconds (you may need to add a bit more oil to pan).

Divide onions among the three circles of dough. Spread marinara sauce over onions, then sprinkle on peppers and mushrooms. Next add tomato-and-garlic mixture. Sprinkle all with fennel, herbs and red pepper flakes. Place each pan (or two if they fit) on a cookie sheet and bake 20 minutes on lowest shelf in oven.

Brush visible crust with oil and continue baking 5 to 10 minutes or until crust is golden brown (or darker if you prefer).

YIELD: 3 8-inch pizzas

"Peppercorn"

4 green bell peppers
4 red bell peppers
2 to 3 large leeks, cleaned
   and trimmed carefully
2 tablespoons corn oil

4 ears corn, with
   kernels cut from cob
2 to 3 green chili peppers
   (optional)
Chopped garlic, to taste

Dice green and red bell peppers. Slice leeks diagonally. In a large wok*, stir-fry** all ingredients, except garlic, in hot oil. Toss in garlic, stir a moment and serve immediately.

YIELD: 2 servings

---

* If your stove will not accommodate a large wok, use a small wok or sauté pan. However, since too much food in too small a pan will steam, not stir-fry, you may want to stir-fry the green and red bell peppers first, then the remainder of the vegetables, adding oil as you need it.

** To stir-fry, heat the oil to hot (a drop of water will spatter and sizzle when dropped into hot oil). Add the vegetables and toss quickly, keeping them moving. In this recipe, the stir-frying should take no longer than 4 minutes, provided you like crunchy vegetables.

Vegetable Fried Rice

2 to 3 leeks cut diagonally, white part only
10 fresh mushrooms and/or 8 dried shiitake mushrooms, soaked
10 snow peas, cleaned
12 to 16 asparagus spears, cut diagonally

1 cup brown rice, uncooked
2 cups water
3 to 4 tablespoons light-colored sesame oil
1 to 2 cloves garlic, minced
2 teaspoons grated fresh ginger

Dice leeks, mushrooms and snow peas into bite-size pieces. Cut asparagus spears into long or short diagonals.

Bring rice and water to a boil, then turn to low and simmer, covered, for about 40 to 45 minutes.

Heat 1 to 2 tablespoons oil in wok or skillet until hot enough for drop of water to sizzle. Stir-fry vegetables quickly, turning and moving them for 1 to 2 minutes or until they are done the way you like them. Cooking time will, of course, depend on how large or small you have cut them.

Toss in garlic and ginger. Add rice, turning quickly and adding more oil if needed. Cook only long enough to make certain rice is hot (about 2 minutes). Serve immediately.

YIELD: 2 servings

Chinese Stir-Fry Vegetables

24 asparagus spears
4 to 5 leeks, well cleaned,
   white part only
30 snow peas
1 teaspoon light-colored
   sesame oil

1 to 2 cloves garlic,
   minced
2 teaspoons grated fresh
   ginger

Cut asparagus spears and leeks diagonally. Remove stems from snow peas.

Sauté or stir-fry vegetables for about 5 minutes in hot oil. Toss in garlic and ginger,* stir a moment. Serve immediately.

YIELD: 2 servings

Variation: Super Veggie Stir-Fry

Try this dish with broccoli, mushrooms (fresh or dried shiitake mushrooms that have been soaked in warm water and stems removed), leeks and pea pods.

Variation: Stir-Fry with Oriental Noodles

Add cooked oriental noodles to your stir-fry, or stir-fry mostly cooked noodles and add red pepper flakes and a few of the above-mentioned vegetables that have been stir-fried first. Bok choy is good in this recipe, and celery is always a reliable choice.

---

* Garlic and ginger may be stir-fried first. This is the traditional method, but the garlic will be bitter. Also, if you want the leeks to be more well done, cook them 3 minutes alone to start.

Tempura Mazel

Tempura is a Japanese dish. Tidbits are dipped in a batter of flour, water and egg yolk, sizzled until golden in hot fat (by all means, use your wok for this if you have one), drained, and artistically arranged and served, usually on a doily-lined flat basket. The consistency of the batter (which must be neither too thick nor too thin) and the temperature of the oil (350°F is just right) are of the utmost importance. Tempura cannot wait; it must go directly from wok to table.

5 asparagus spears, cut diagonally into 2- to 3-inch-long pieces

1 to 2 large carrots, sliced diagonally into 1/4-inch thick pieces

10 green beans, ends trimmed

2 small zucchini, cut into thick sticks

1 bell pepper, cut into strips

6 dried shiitake mushrooms, soaked in warm water

6 large parsley sprigs, stems removed

4 sheets nori seaweed, cut into quarters (available in Asian markets)

1 1/2 quarts safflower oil (more if using sauté pan)

Clean and cut vegetables; make certain they are dry.

Batter:

2 1/4 cups flour

Ice water

3 egg yolks

Place flour in a large bowl. Gradually add ice water, mixing with a whisk, until mixture is the consistency of heavy cream. Beat yolks; whisk into flour-water mixture.

Heat oil to 350°F in wok or large deep pan. (Caution: never fill a pan more than ⅓ full with oil.) Dip vegetables into batter and fry until golden (1 to 2 minutes). Do not crowd pan. Drain on paper towels and serve immediately.

YIELD: 5 to 6 servings

WELL OILED: *It's important to know approximately how much oil your pans require for proper frying. If a pan is heavy and well seasoned, you can cook with less oil. If the oil is hot and you refrain from adding too many ingredients to the pan at one time, you can get away with using less oil. Start with less oil than the recipe calls for, adding more only if you need it to keep the food from sticking to the pan. For Mexican flavoring, use canola oil; for Italian, use olive oil.*

Chilies Mazel

6 fresh green New Mexico chilies	1 egg yolk
1 recipe **Mazel "Cheese" Mexican**, warmed	Sesame oil for deep frying (about 1½ quarts)
Ice water	1 recipe **Hot and Spicy Salsa Mazel**
¾ cup flour	

Slice chilies open lengthwise, just enough to stuff with Mazel Cheese Mexican. Clean out seeds and pith. Stuff with Mazel Cheese mixture and set aside.

Gently whisk enough ice water into flour to make it about the consistency of heavy cream. Beat egg yolk with a fork, then whisk into batter.

Heat oil to 350°F. Dip each chili into batter. Cook in oil until golden (1 to 2 minutes).* Drain on paper towels.

Serve cooked salsa over chilies.

YIELD: 2 servings

CHILIES: *Today the five domesticated species of chili account for over 2,000 varieties ranging in size from ¼ inch to more than a foot long. All are members of the nightshade family along with tomatoes, potatoes and eggplants.*

---

* The timing on deep frying is difficult to pinpoint. Variables include size of pan, amount of oil used, temperature of oil, desired color of finished product, etc. Do not crowd pan. An instant-read cooking thermometer is the best way to gauge the oil's temperature. If you do not have a thermometer, try this trick: Place a sugar-cube-size piece of white bread in the hot oil and note how long it takes to turn golden brown. The oil is right (about 350°F) if the bread browns in 1 minute.

Mazel Mex

2½ cups cold water
1¼ cups cornmeal
Generous dash cayenne
   pepper and/or cinnamon
3 onions, coarsely chopped
⅔ tablespoon corn oil
8 large tomatoes, coarsely
   chopped*
1 to 2 fresh New Mexico
   chilies or jalapeño peppers,
   peeled and coarsely
   chopped

1 to 2 cloves garlic,
   minced
1 tablespoon chopped
   fresh cilantro
1 tablespoon chopped
   fresh parsley

Combine water, cornmeal and cayenne and/or cinnamon. Add to saucepan and cook, stirring frequently,
over medium heat for 5 to 8 minutes.

Remove mixture from heat and pat evenly onto
bottom of 8 x 12-inch casserole.

In large pan, cook onions in corn oil over medium
heat until translucent and fairly soft (10 to 15 minutes). Add tomatoes, chilies and garlic; cook 2 to 3
minutes.

Pour mixture over cornmeal base and bake in
350°F oven for 20 to 25 minutes.

To serve, sprinkle with cilantro and parsley.

YIELD: 2 servings

---

* Although taste is bitter if tomatoes are unpeeled, the peels are an important
aid to digestion.

CHILIES: *The hot in hot chilies is caused by capsaicin (cap-SAY-i-sin), an odorless, colorless and flavorless chemical found in the seeds and internal membranes of the pepper. Capsaicin is so potent that a single drop placed in a million drops of water still packs a noticeable bite.*

The chilies used in the recipes in this book are New Mexico chilies and jalapeños. The New Mexico variety is a mild chili with a peppery flavor and mild fruitiness much like a bell pepper. Jalapeños are the most popular chili in the United States. They are only moderately hot by chili standards, but care must be taken in handling them.

Mazel Enchiladas

¼ cup corn oil
6 to 8 corn tortillas
1 recipe **Hot and Spicy Salsa Mazel**

2 recipes **Mazel "Cheese" Mexican***
1 recipe **Fresh Mexican Salsa**

Heat corn oil in large skillet. Using tongs, dip corn tortillas in hot corn oil, then into cooked salsa.

Place in a large baking dish, fill with Mazel Cheese Mexican and roll into enchiladas, arranging in orderly rows. Cover with Hot and Spicy Salsa Mazel. Bake uncovered at 350°F for 15 to 20 minutes. Serve with Fresh Mexican Salsa.

YIELD: 2 servings

Variation 1: Add 1 bunch fresh spinach, cooked and chopped, to Mazel Cheese Mexican.

Variation 2: Add 1 tablespoon fresh mixed chives and parsley to Mazel Cheese Mexican.

Variation 3: Use one recipe Mazel Cheese Mexican and 1½ to 2 cups sour cream rather than two recipes Mazel Cheese Mexican.

---

* Depending on size of tortillas and how you fill them, you may wind up with a bit of extra filling. If so, add it to the casserole or reserve it for another use—but better too much than too little.

Fried Matzo Mazel

½ stick unsalted butter
3 onions, sliced or
  chopped

6 sheets unsalted matzo,
  soaked in water and
  squeezed

Heat butter in skillet. Add onions and sauté until brown and crispy. Add matzo and cook until golden.
YIELD: 2 servings

Zucchini Pancakes

You can substitute carrots for zucchini.

2 pounds zucchini
 (or carrots)
1 onion, minced
3 egg yolks, lightly
 beaten
1 cup whole-wheat
 pastry flour (or 1 cup
 unbleached flour)
1 teaspoon double-acting
 baking powder (low-
 sodium variety available
 at health food stores)

Freshly ground black
 pepper, to taste
Freshly ground or grated
 nutmeg
1 tablespoon minced fresh
 basil (or $\frac{1}{2}$ tablespoon
 dried)
4 teaspoons olive oil
Safflower oil for frying
Sour cream (optional)

Wash and grate zucchini. Combine with onion. Stir in egg yolks, flour, baking powder, pepper, nutmeg and basil. Stir in olive oil and allow batter to rest for 15 minutes.

Fill a large frying pan with safflower oil and place on medium heat. Drop batter into hot oil and flatten into pancakes. Brown both sides. Drain on paper towels and keep warm.

Continue with the rest of the batter, adding oil as necessary. Serve with sour cream. (They are also delicious served plain.)

YIELD: 4 to 5 servings

Asparagus in Garlic-Herb Bread Crumbs

Almost any other vegetable can be substituted for asparagus.

1 bunch asparagus
    (about 2 dozen)
7 tablespoons butter
1 cup **Bread Crumbs**
1 teaspoon dried thyme
    (or 2 teaspoons fresh)
1 teaspoon minced fresh
    basil

1 teaspoon dried oregano
1 teaspoon minced fresh
    Italian parsley
Small pinch grated fresh
    ginger (optional)
3 cloves garlic, minced

Select firm, fresh asparagus. The tips should be tight and closed.

Wash asparagus, cut off the woody ends of the stalks and trim spears to equal length. Tie together in 2 bunches and cook in boiling water for about 10 minutes or until just fork-tender. Drain and set aside.

In a sauté pan, melt butter and add bread crumbs, sautéing until lightly browned. Add herbs, ginger and garlic, stirring gently to combine.

Pour over asparagus and serve.

YIELD: 4 servings

FRESH IS BETTER: *You may substitute dried herbs for fresh, but they will not produce the same results. An herb's flavor is concentrated in volatile oils found in the leaves. Drying concentrates the flavor by breaking down the plant cell structure and releasing the oils. Initially, dried herbs are more potent than fresh. But over time, the oils evaporate and dried herbs slowly lose their flavor.*

Vegetarian Antipasto

The freshness and appearance of the vegetables in this dish are very important. Choose the vegetables with particular care.

1 pound carrots
1 large bunch broccoli
   (minimum 1 pound)
1 large cauliflower
1/2 small, tight head
   red cabbage
3 large artichokes
4 small red peppers
   (long, spicy variety of
   red Italian peppers)
2 firm, small zucchini

1 bulb fennel (if unavailable,
   use fennel seeds)
4 tomatoes
1 large red onion
1 pound fresh mushrooms
1/4 cup rice vinegar
2 cloves garlic, minced
2 tablespoons shallot,
   minced
Freshly ground black
   pepper, to taste
1/2 cup olive oil

Wash and scrape carrots and cut into 3-inch-long julienne. Break broccoli and cauliflower into bite-sized florets and wash. Shred cabbage. Cut outside leaves and large stems from artichokes.

Place artichokes in a large pot of boiling water and simmer until still firm but tender when pierced at the bottom. Drain, refresh with cold water to retain color, remove all leaves and choke, and cut bottoms into large chunks. Carrots, broccoli and cauliflower should be cooked separately in simmering water until just fork-tender. Refresh all with cold water immediately after cooking.

Place shredded cabbage in a bowl and pour boiling water over it. Drain after 3 minutes; refresh with cold water immediately.

Char peppers over a burner on high; cool, peel off skin, and seed. Cut into thin strips.

Peel and slice zucchini into julienne.

Pull apart the fennel bulb and slice into long, thin strips. (Discard stalks, or use to flavor soup.)

Slice tomatoes into wedges and remove seeds.

Slice red onion into thin rounds.

Prepare antipasto platter, arranging the vegetables in a circular pattern from the outside toward the center, with the larger pieces on the outside. Be sure to contrast the colors as well as the sizes.

Remove stems from mushrooms and slice caps paper-thin. Sprinkle mushrooms over all.

Sprinkle vinegar over antipasto. Season with garlic, shallot and pepper; toss lightly. Drizzle with oil and serve.

YIELD: 4 servings

CARROTS: *Carrots and other similar vegetables should be well scrubbed, but do not peel them—many valuable nutrients lie close to the skin.*

Pizza con Cipolle
(Pizza with Onions)

A Sicilian-style pizza with onions, garlic and herbs. It's delicious!

Dough:

1 cake fresh yeast (or 1 package active dry yeast)	*1½ cups tepid water*
⅓ cup tepid water	*2 cups whole-wheat flour*
	2 cups bread flour or unbleached flour

Filling:

6 tablespoons unsalted butter	*½ cup fresh Italian parsley, chopped*
½ cup olive oil	*3 tablespoons fresh oregano*
8 onions, sliced paper-thin	*Freshly ground black pepper, to taste*
8 garlic cloves, minced	
1 cup bread crumbs	

Dough:

Place yeast in ⅓ cup tepid water (90° to 100°F). Stir to dissolve. Mix in a food processor for 10 seconds. Add 1½ cups tepid water and again process for 10 seconds. Then, by level cupfuls, add the flours to processor, running for 30 seconds after each addition, until absorbed. When adding final cup, do not put in full amount at once. (Flour absorbs moisture differently at different times. Add it gradually until you achieve the texture described below.) Knead the dough in the processor for about 1 minute or until it begins to ball up and accumulate on the top of the blade and is a somewhat sticky, homogeneous mass. Flour your hands, remove the dough to a floured surface and knead for a minute or so by hand.

Form into a large, fat pancake shape, place on a lightly floured plate, sprinkle the top with flour and cover with plastic wrap. Refrigerate for about 6 hours before making pizza.

Filling:

In a large sauté pan or skillet, melt 3 tablespoons butter with $1/4$ cup olive oil, saving $1/4$ cup for assembly of pizza. When heated, add onion slices and half the minced garlic. Over low heat, cook until onions are completely wilted but not brown (20 to 25 minutes). In a smaller sauté pan, melt remaining 3 tablespoons of butter, add bread crumbs and sauté until golden. Add remaining garlic, parsley and oregano to the bread crumbs, mix thoroughly, and cook until flavors are blended. Grind black pepper over all. Mix and set aside until ready to assemble pizza.

Assembly of Pizza:

Preheat oven to 450°F. Remove dough from refrigerator and allow to rest at room temperature for 15 minutes. Meanwhile, grease a large jelly-roll pan (11 x 18 inches), preferably the heavy black variety, with 1 tablespoon olive oil. Using a rolling pin on a floured work surface, roll dough into a rectangle approximately the same size as the pan. Place the dough in the pan and with your hands work it into the corners of the pan, making it higher at the sides than in the middle. Bake at 450°F for 15 to 20 minutes, until risen and lightly browned.

Remove from oven. Spread onions over crust, top with bread crumb mixture, sprinkle with remaining olive oil (about ¼ cup), return to oven and bake 10 to 15 minutes longer or until browned and cooked through. Cut in large squares and serve.

YIELD: 5 to 6 servings

Variation: Handmade Dough

To make dough by hand, place yeast in ⅓ cup tepid water and stir to dissolve. Place 2 cups of whole-wheat and 2 cups of white flour in a large bowl and combine. Make a well in the center and add dissolved yeast and 1½ cups water. Using your index finger, stir the flour into the liquid. Work the mixture together well, turn out onto a floured work surface and knead, pushing and turning the dough exactly as you would if you were making bread. If the dough becomes sticky as you knead, sprinkle on a bit more flour. The dough is ready when it is smooth and elastic. Kneading to this point should take approximately 10 minutes. Proceed with recipe above.

STORING HERBS: *If properly stored in airtight containers, crushed or ground dry herbs can maintain flavor for up to six months; whole-leaf herbs will remain flavorful for up to a year.*

Oven Fries

2-pound mix of the follow-
    ing vegetables: potatoes,
    carrots, jicama
3 egg whites
$\frac{1}{2}$ teaspoon paprika

$\frac{1}{4}$ teaspoon cayenne
    pepper (optional)
1 tablespoon chopped
    fresh parsley

Slice vegetables into $\frac{1}{2}$ x 2-inch slices and allow to dry thoroughly. In a small bowl mix egg whites, spices and parsley, whisking until frothy. Coat vegetables thoroughly and lay $\frac{1}{2}$ inch apart on an ungreased baking sheet.

Bake in a 350°F oven for 20 minutes or until "fries" are crispy outside but still soft inside. Serve with **Mazel Ketchup**.

YIELD: 4 to 6 servings

Asian Noodles with Peas and Peppers

6 ounces buckwheat
   noodles
3 tablespoons sesame oil
2 cloves garlic, minced
1 tablespoon fresh ginger
½ pound snow peas,
   cleaned with strings
   removed
1 large red pepper,
   seeded and julienned

1 large green pepper,
   seeded and julienned
3 green onions, thinly
   sliced
1 tablespoon sesame oil
   (amber-colored, Asian-
   style)
1 tablespoon fresh cilantro

Cook noodles according to directions on the package, drain and set aside. In a wok or large nonstick sauté pan, heat sesame oil until hot. Add garlic and ginger. Cook until light brown, stirring constantly. Add peas and peppers, and cook until crisp tender (2 to 3 minutes). Add green onions and cook for a few more seconds.

In a large bowl combine cooked vegetables and noodles, add sesame oil, and cilantro. Toss well and serve immediately.

YIELD: 2 servings

Spinach-Stuffed Tomatoes

2 large tomatoes
1 pound fresh spinach,
    washed and stems
    removed

1 recipe **Béchamel Sauce**
Bread Crumbs

Prepare béchamel sauce and set aside. Steam spinach until tender; drain well and allow to cool. Meanwhile, cut holes in tops of tomatoes, and scoop out seeds and pulp.

Preheat oven to 350°F. When spinach is cooled, chop coarsely. Combine spinach with béchamel sauce and stir to combine thoroughly. Stuff spinach mixture into reserved tomatoes and place in a baking dish.

Bake tomatoes for 20 minutes or until heated through. Garnish with bread crumbs.

YIELD: 2 servings

Spicy Thai Noodles

4 cloves garlic
1 tablespoon chile oil
2 tablespoons sesame oil
  (amber-colored, Asian-
  style)
1 tablespoon fresh ginger,
  grated
1 tablespoon rice vinegar
2 tablespoons fresh
  cilantro, coarsely chopped

½ pound pea pods
½ pound asparagus
½ pound broccoli
1 pound spaghetti
1 carrot, grated
1 cucumber, peeled and
  diced
1 bunch green onions,
  chopped, including some
  green

In a food processor, process the garlic first then add chili oil, sesame oil, ginger and vinegar. Process until smooth. Scrape the sauce into a large bowl and add the cilantro. Stir to combine.

Blanch the pea pods, asparagus and broccoli, taking care to retain their bright green color and crunchy texture. Rinse in cold water. Allow to drain.

Cook spaghetti per package directions until al dente. Drain and immediately transfer to large bowl containing sauce. Add pea pods, asparagus, broccoli and carrots, and mix well.

Arrange pasta on serving platter and garnish with cucumber and green onions. Serve warm or chill and serve as a luncheon salad.

YIELD: 4 to 6 servings

ELEVEN

Beefing It Up

Butterflied Leg of Lamb

¹/₄ cup Dijon-style salt-free mustard (or 2 tablespoons dry mustard mixed with 2 teaspoons **Fonds Brun**)
2 cloves garlic, mashed
1 teaspoon grated fresh ginger
1 tablespoon dried rosemary, crushed

Freshly ground black pepper, to taste
2 tablespoons olive oil
1 leg of lamb, boned and butterflied (ask your butcher to do this for you)

In a small mixing bowl, combine mustard, garlic, ginger, rosemary and pepper. Drop by drop, whisk in oil until marinade has a mayonnaise-like consistency.

Spread marinade on lamb and allow to marinate all day if possible.

Preheat broiler until hot. Broil lamb 7 minutes on each side for rare; increase time if you prefer your meat more well done.

You may grill lamb on an open barbecue for about 10 minutes on each side for rare, increase time for a more well done meat.

YIELD: 6 servings

SHAKING SALT: *If you miss the flavor of salt in any dish, compensate by adding more fresh chopped herbs and garlic or one of the flavorful salt substitutes found at supermarkets and health food stores (Mrs. Dash is my favorite). Be sure to read the label carefully and check for added sodium. Freshly ground pepper can also add flavor to your dishes. Be certain to buy peppercorns in a store where there is a fast turnover of this product; stale pepper has a bite but little flavor.*

Steak au Poivre

2 tablespoons black or   3 tablespoons oil
green peppercorns,   1 cup heavy cream
crushed
4 1½-inch-thick
strip steaks

Scatter peppercorns on a large plate and coat
steaks on both sides by pressing them onto peppercorns.

In a large sauté pan, heat the oil until nearly smok-
ing. Add steaks and sauté over medium-high heat
until rare (about 5 minutes on each side). Set aside
to keep warm.

Pour off the fat in the pan, add cream, increase
heat to high and boil cream until it thickens somewhat. Pour over steaks and serve.

YIELD: 4 servings

Veau Poêlé à la Moutarde
(Casserole-Roasted Veal with Mustard)

2 pounds boned shoulder
  of veal
3 garlic cloves, minced
1 teaspoon dried rosemary,
  crushed
2 teaspoons dried thyme
  Freshly ground black
  pepper, to taste

2 tablespoons olive oil
3 tablespoons butter
⅔ cup veal stock or
  Fonds Brun (additional
  ½ to ¾ cup if needed)
2 tablespoons chopped
  shallot
¼ cup Dijon-style
  salt-free mustard
½ cup heavy cream

Open roast and lay flat. Sprinkle with garlic, rosemary, thyme and pepper. Roll and tie roast with kitchen twine.

In a large, covered, heavy saucepan or casserole, heat oil and 2 tablespoons butter over medium-high heat until foaming. Add veal to pan and brown meat well on all sides. Pour stock over roast, reduce heat, cover and cook until fork-tender. During the cooking, turn meat to make sure it roasts evenly. Add more stock if pan juices run clear when veal is pierced.

Remove roast from pan and set aside to keep warm. If no pan juices remain, stir in about ½ cup stock, raise heat and scrape up the bits at the bottom of the pan with a wooden spoon. Add remaining butter. When melted, add shallots and cook until wilted (4 to 5 minutes). Whisk in mustard. Raise flame, pour in cream, and heat until bubbling and thickened slightly. Pour over roast and serve.

YIELD: 4 to 6 servings

Flank Steak Provençal

2 tablespoons sesame oil	1/4 teaspoon black pepper
2 tablespoons chopped fresh parsley	1 tablespoon minced fresh thyme
2 cloves garlic, minced	2 pounds flank steak

In a small bowl combine oil, parsley, garlic, thyme and pepper. Mix well. Rub half of the herb mixture on one side of the steak. Reserve the remainder. Let steak stand at room temperature for 1 hour.

Preheat broiler. Place steak, oiled side up, on broiler pan. Broil 4 inches from heat for about 5 minutes. Turn steak and brush with remaining mixture. Broil until desired doneness. Serve with mustard butter.

Mustard butter:

1/2 cup softened unsalted butter	2 tablespoons stone-ground mustard

Combine all ingredients in a small bowl and mix until well combined

YIELD: 4 servings

Curried Pork Tenderloin

1 pork tenderloin	2 tablespoons curry powder
(8 to 10 ounces)	2 cups plain yogurt
2 tablespoons sesame oil	2 hard boiled eggs,
2 cloves garlic	chopped

Slice tenderloin into 8 to 10 medallions.

In a small bowl combine sesame oil, garlic, curry powder, and yogurt. Reserve half of the mixture for garnish, pour the other half into a shallow dish. Add the pork, coat thoroughly cover dish and refrigerate. Marinate 30 minutes, turning once.

Preheat oven to 350°F. Remove pork from the yogurt mixture and place in a baking dish. Cook pork for 30 to 40 minutes or until meat is opaque and still tender. Baste occasionally with the left over marinade.

When pork is done, remove medallions to individual plates (3 to 4 per serving) and garnish with reserved curry mixture and chopped hard-boiled eggs.

YIELD: 3 to 4 servings

TWELVE

The Open Sea

Cold Seafood Salad

You will need about 3½ pounds of seafood (weighed in the shell except for scallops). Choose any combination of shrimp, scallops, crab or lobster.

2½ tablespoons
  unsalted butter
¼ cup minced shallot
1 pound shrimp, peeled
  and veins removed
½ pound sea scallops,
  washed and cut in half
½ cup **Court Bouillon**

1 live 1-pound lobster
1 live 1-pound crab
3 tablespoons minced fresh
  tarragon (or 1½
  tablespoons dried)
1 cup **Protein Mayonnaise**

Melt 2 tablespoons butter in a medium sauté pan. Sprinkle shallots over bottom of pan. Rinse seafood and pat dry. Place shrimp and scallops over the shallots and add ½ cup court bouillon. With remaining ½ tablespoon butter, butter a sheet of waxed paper and lay it buttered side down over ingredients in pan. Put lid on pan and place over low heat. Cook 10 to 15 minutes, or until bouillon comes to a slow simmer. Strain, cool and refrigerate.

Bring a large pan (big enough to accommodate the live lobster and crab) of water to a vigorous boil. Add whole lobster and crab, cover and cook over medium heat for 5 to 10 minutes, depending on their size. DO NOT use cooked crab legs, such as King crab or snow crab. These species are typically brine frozen and contain high levels of sodium. Plan on 5 to 7 minutes of cooking time for the first pound and half that time for each additional pound. Drain, cool and refrigerate.

To assemble the salad: Crack lobster and crab, removing meat in chunks and cutting it into 1-inch cubes. Place in large bowl. Add shrimp and scallops.

Whisk the tarragon into the mayonnaise and toss with seafood. Refrigerate until ready to serve.

YIELD: 4 servings

Sole en Papillote, Crème à l'Échalote
(Sole in an Envelope, Shallot Cream)

Cooked in aluminum foil or parchment paper, the fish steams in its own juices. The flavor is fresh and intense.

6 sprigs Italian parsley
3 shallots, minced
2 cloves garlic, minced
1½ pounds lemon sole, divided into 4 servings
4 tablespoons unsalted butter

Freshly ground white pepper, to taste
*2 cups **Crème à l'Échalote** (substitute fish stock or chicken stock)*

Preheat oven to 500°F.

Cut sheets of aluminum foil into 4 large heart shapes of approximately 15 inches in width and height. Oil entire piece of foil, fold in half along center seam of the heart and open again. Repeat the procedure for all 4 hearts.

Divide parsley and distribute equally on half of each heart. Cover parsley with shallots and garlic. Top with a portion of sole, 1 tablespoon butter and white pepper.

Place the baking dish in which the papillotes will cook in the oven to preheat.

Fold over the other half of each heart so its edges match those of the first half. Starting at the bottom point, begin folding foil over on itself so that bit by bit you make a $\frac{1}{2}$-inch border all the way to the top. Pinch the edges tightly to make sure you have an airtight packet of foil in which the fish can steam.

Place the foil envelopes in the preheated baking dish. Bake for 5 minutes.

Serve fish still enclosed in the foil, permitting each person to cut open his or her own papillote and enjoy the wonderful aroma that arises from it.

Serve with crème à l'échalote.

YIELD: 4 servings

Filets de Saumon à l'Oseille
(Salmon Fillets with Sorrel)

4 cups sorrel leaves,
  tightly packed
  (approximately 1 pound)
4 tablespoons unsalted
  butter
2 shallots, minced
2 large fillets of fresh
  salmon (approximately
  3 to 4 pounds)

Freshly ground white
  pepper, to taste
1 quart **Court Bouillon**
  (approximately)
1½ cups heavy cream

Wash, dry and remove the heavy stems from sorrel; cut leaves into long, thin strips.

Preheat oven to 375°F.

Choose a large, low-sided gratin dish or an enameled-iron roasting pan to poach fillets in the oven. The dish must be ovenproof.

Grease the dish with 1 tablespoon of butter. Sprinkle in shallots and add fillets. Season with white pepper and add just enough court bouillon to nearly cover fillets.

Place a piece of buttered wax paper over fillets, buttered side down, and bring to a low simmer on top of stove.

Place in oven and cook for 10 to 12 minutes or until fish is still moist but separates easily when poked with a fork.

Drain fillets and place poaching liquid in a heavy

saucepan on top of stove. Keep fish warm while preparing the sauce.

Bring poaching liquid to a boil over high heat and reduce by about one-third. Add cream and, still over high heat, continue to reduce until thickened. Remove from heat, add sorrel; cook for just 1 minute more. Remove from heat and stir in remaining butter.

Pour sauce over fillets and serve.

YIELD: 4 servings

Moules à la Marinière
(Steamed Mussels)

4 quarts fresh mussels,
  beards removed, soaked
  and scrubbed clean
3 cloves garlic with husks
  left on, crushed
½ cup chopped shallot
1 bay leaf
4 sprigs fresh thyme
  (or 2 teaspoons dried)
4 sprigs fresh Italian
  parsley

Freshly ground black
  pepper, to taste
¼ teaspoon red
  pepper flakes
1 cup fish stock or
  Fumet de Poisson, or
  ¾ cup water mixed
  with ¼ cup clam juice
2 tablespoons minced fresh
  Italian parsley

Place mussels, garlic, shallot, bay leaf, thyme, parsley sprigs, pepper and red pepper flakes in a large, heavy saucepan. Pour in fish stock, cover and bring to a boil.

Steam mussels over medium heat until they open (5 to 6 minutes). Discard any that do not open.

Place mussels in soup bowls and pour cooking liquid over them. Top with minced parsley and serve.

YIELD: 4 servings

Moules Farcies à la Crème, à l'Anis et au Thym
(Stuffed Mussels with Cream, Anise and Thyme)

4 quarts mussels, steamed open as in **Moules à la Marinière**	2 cloves garlic, minced
	2 shallots, minced
	½ cup heavy cream
2 tablespoons unsalted butter	Pinch of thyme
	Pinch of star anise

Steam mussels for approximately 5 minutes or until open. Discard those that don't open. Remove mussels from shells. Reserve half the shells to stuff. Place mussels on work surface and chop into small pieces.

Melt butter in sauté pan; add garlic and shallots. Cook until wilted. Add mussels, cream, thyme and anise. Raise heat and reduce mixture quickly by about half.

Fill mussel shells with mixture, place on cookie sheet and brown for 3 minutes under broiler. Serve immediately.

YIELD: 3 to 4 servings

Herbed Red Snapper

Black pepper, to taste
⅓ cup **Protein Mayonnaise**
½ tablespoon Dijon mus-
  tard
1 cup loosely packed fresh

  parsley
1 tablespoon chopped fresh
  tarragon leaves
1½ pounds red snapper
  fillets

Preheat oven to 400°F.

In small bowl, combine pepper, mayonnaise, mustard and chopped herbs. Mix to combine well. Set aside to allow flavors to blend.

Wash snapper fillets and pat dry with a towel. Lightly brush one side of fillets with sesame oil. Place oiled side down in a glass baking dish. Spoon herb-and-mayonnaise mixture over fillets. Place pan in oven and bake until opaque in center (about 8 to 10 minutes per inch of thickness).

YIELD: 4 servings

Basil-Tarragon Steamed Salmon

1 5- to 6-pound salmon,
   cleaned
2 tablespoons sesame oil
Freshly ground black
   pepper, to taste

2 tablespoons fresh
   tarragon, minced
2 tablespoons fresh basil,
   minced

Rinse salmon in cool water and pat dry with a paper towel inside and out. Rub inside cavity with sesame oil and season with pepper. Evenly distribute fresh minced herbs inside the cavity. Place salmon on large piece of foil and wrap, making sure to seal ends tightly.

Place foil package on a hot barbeque grill and cook approximately 30 minutes, turning carefully after 10 minutes. Slice foil open, being careful to avoid hot steam when it escapes. Remove foil and transfer fish to a serving platter. Garnish with fresh herb sprigs.

YIELD: 4 servings

Grilled Mahimahi

1½- to 2-pound mahimahi
  filet

Marinade:

³/₄ cup plain yogurt   2 teaspoons crushed red
1 teaspoon cumin   pepper
1 teaspoon nutmeg   Coarsely ground black
1 teaspoon ground clove   pepper, to taste

Rinse fish in cool water and pat dry with a paper towel. Cut into four equal portions.

In a small bowl, combine marinade ingredients and mix to combine. Place whole fish in a heavyweight resealable plastic bag and coat thoroughly with marinade. Place in refrigerator and allow to marinate for 30 minutes.

Remove from marinade and grill fish over hot indirect heat, until flesh is opaque (about 30 minutes) turning once. Transfer to a large serving platter.

YIELD: 4 servings

THIRTEEN

❧

Fowl Play

Broiled Chicken
with Herb-Mustard Coating

2 tablespoons dry
  mustard
2 tablespoons chicken
  stock or **Fonds de
  Volaille**
2 tablespoons fresh
  tarragon (1 tablespoon
  dried) or 1 tablespoon
  fresh rosemary (1½
  teaspoons dried)

1 teaspoon grated fresh
  ginger
Freshly ground white
  pepper, to taste
Freshly ground or grated
  nutmeg, to taste
1 broiling chicken, cut into
  serving-size pieces

In a small bowl combine dry mustard and chicken
stock. Add tarragon or rosemary, ginger, white pepper
and nutmeg; mix to a paste.

Coat chicken pieces with herb-mustard mixture.
Allow to marinate for 1 hour.

Preheat oven to 350°F.

Bake chicken for 30 minutes. Transfer to broiler,
skin side up, and broil for 8 to 10 minutes or until
lightly browned. Serve immediately.

YIELD: 3 to 4 servings

FRESH HERBS: *Fresh herbs should be stored in your refrigerator. Place bunches upright in a container filled with an inch or so of water. Smaller quantities can be placed in a plastic bag or moistened paper towels and stored in your refrigerator's crisper.*

Coq à l'Ail
(Chicken with Garlic)

Until you try this, you will never believe how sweet garlic can taste with chicken. It's sensational!

4 to 6 tablespoons oil
2 large roasting chickens
(about 4 pounds each),
cut into serving-size pieces
4 tablespoons unsalted
butter
1 cup minced shallot
2 tablespoons dried tarragon
2 large heads of garlic
(or 3 small), separated
into cloves, husks left on
(at least 30 small cloves)

Freshly ground black
pepper, to taste
10 sprigs fresh Italian
parsley
1 cup chicken stock or
Fonds de Volaille

Preheat oven to 375°F.

In a large, cast-iron or heavy casserole, heat 4 table-spoons oil until very hot. Meanwhile, wipe chicken parts with paper towel until they are completely dry. Brown chicken in the oil, skin side first, then turn to brown on other side. Remove chicken and set aside. Continue until all pieces are browned, adding more oil if necessary. When browning is completed, discard remaining fat.

Melt butter in the casserole used to brown chicken. Add shallot, chicken, tarragon, garlic, pepper and parsley. Pour the chicken stock over all.

Cover the casserole with a tight-fitting lid and place in preheated oven for 1 hour and 15 minutes.

When chicken is ready, remove to a serving platter. Strain pan juices to serve with chicken. Remove garlic cloves from the strained-out herbs and scatter garlic over chicken. Eat the softened garlic by slipping it from its husk and spreading it on chicken.

YIELD: 4 servings

Suprêmes de Volaille à l'Estragon

(Chicken Breasts with Tarragon)

3 teaspoons unsalted
  butter
6 chicken breast halves,
  skinned and boned
¼ cup minced shallot
¾ cup chicken stock or
  Fonds de Volaille
2 teaspoons minced
  fresh tarragon (or
  1 tablespoon dried)

Freshly ground white
  pepper, to taste
½ cup heavy cream
A few sprigs fresh
  tarragon

Melt butter in a large sauté pan. Add chicken and sauté on both sides over low to medium heat, just until chicken whitens and loses its raw pink color.

Sprinkle shallot over chicken, pour in the stock, and add tarragon and pepper. Cover and gently poach for 5 minutes.

Remove cover and raise heat to high. Scraping bottom of pan with a wooden spoon, reduce stock until only about ¼ cup remains. Pour in cream and, still over high heat, continue reducing sauce until thickened.

Remove chicken to a warm serving platter, pour sauce over it, garnish with a few tarragon sprigs and serve immediately.

YIELD: 4 servings

Quenelles de Volaille
(Chicken Quenelles)

Light as air and delicious as they are, quenelles are even more of a treat when topped with a sauce or served in a flavorful chicken consommé.

*1 pound chicken breasts,
  skinned and boned
1½ cups heavy cream
Freshly ground white
  pepper, to taste*

*Freshly ground or grated
  nutmeg, to taste
1 egg yolk*

Place chicken and cream in the freezer until well chilled (about 15 minutes).

Cut chicken into cubes and place in a food processor. Add pepper and nutmeg; process for 30 seconds.

Add egg yolk and gently blend it with the chicken. Process for 5 seconds.

With the machine running, add heavy cream in a thin stream.

Transfer mixture to a bowl and refrigerate for 1 hour.

Butter an oval gratin dish large enough to accommodate all quenelles in a single layer.

Shape quenelles with two large soup spoons. Scoop up a spoonful of the mixture in one spoon, then round and shape it with another spoon dipped first into very hot water. As you complete each one, gently place it in the gratin dish. Continue until you have used up all the quenelle mixture.

Bring approximately 7 cups of water to a boil. Ladle water gently over quenelles in the gratin dish to just cover. Place a piece of buttered wax paper that has been cut to the shape of the dish over quenelles (place buttered side down). Bring to a simmer on top of the stove and simmer very gently for 5 minutes. Turn quenelles over gently, replace wax paper and continue poaching for another 5 minutes. Remove and drain on paper towels.

Serve in chicken broth, with **Crème à l'Échalote**, or an herb or butter sauce.

YIELD: 4 servings

Pâté de Foies de Volaille
(Chicken Liver Pâté)

2 tablespoons minced
  shallot
1 tablespoon minced
  garlic
2 tablespoons unsalted
  butter
1 pound chicken livers
¼ cup chicken stock
  (**Fonds de Volaille**)
  or veal stock (**Fonds Brun**)

¼ cup heavy cream
Generous grating of fresh
  nutmeg
2 teaspoons fresh thyme
  (or 1 teaspoon dried)
Freshly ground white
  pepper, to taste
½ cup unsalted butter,
  melted

Sauté the shallot and garlic in 2 tablespoons butter until wilted. While shallots and garlic are cooking, pick over livers to remove membranes.

Add livers to pan and brown quickly on outside, but do not cook through.

Remove from pan and set aside to cool slightly.

Add stock to pan. Raise heat and reduce by half.

Place sautéed livers and reduced liquid in a food processor. Add cream and seasonings; process until pureed and smooth.

Add melted butter and process for 5 seconds.

Distribute among individual ramekins and chill.

YIELD: 4 to 6 servings

QUALITY CHECK: *You can check the potency of dried or fresh herbs by crumbling a small amount between your fingers. The odor should be clear and strong.*

Terrine de Volaille
(Terrine of Chicken)

A good dish for entertaining, this terrine should be made two days ahead of time to allow the flavors to develop.

2 pounds chicken
   breasts, boneless
5 egg whites
Freshly ground white
   pepper, to taste
Freshly grated nutmeg,
   to taste
1/4 teaspoon powdered sage

1/8 teaspoon ground
   cloves
3 tablespoons fresh
   tarragon (or 1 1/2 to
   2 tablespoons dried)
1 1/2 cups heavy cream,
   ice cold

Preheat oven to 350°F.

Place half of chicken breasts in a food processor. Process until chicken becomes a gummy paste. With processor running, slowly add half of egg whites. Add half of herbs and spices. With processor running, slowly pour in half of cream.

Remove mixture from processor and repeat with remaining half of ingredients. Combine both halves in a large bowl and mix thoroughly.

Butter a 1 1/2-quart terrine and fill with chicken mixture. Cover terrine with aluminum foil and place in a bain-marie (or double-boiler), making certain that the boiling water comes two-thirds of the way up the sides of the terrine.

Bake for 45 minutes to 1 hour. Terrine is done when a knife inserted near the center comes out clean. Cool and refrigerate.

YIELD: 4 to 6 servings

Eggs Benedictless

2 eggs
2 tablespoons unsalted
  butter
2 thick-cut slices
  Canadian bacon

³/₄ cup **Hollandaise Sauce**
Pinch of cayenne pepper

In a small saucepan, poach eggs for 3 minutes. While poaching, melt butter in a small sauté pan. When butter foams, add Canadian bacon and cook until lightly browned on one side; turn and finish browning.

Place Canadian bacon on a warmed platter. Top each slice with a poached egg and hollandaise sauce.

Add cayenne and serve immediately.

YIELD: 1 serving

Chicken Parmesan

This easy and delicious dish works equally well with veal.

2 whole chicken breasts,
  divided in half, bone
  and skin removed
1 tablespoon paprika
1 tablespoon onion or
  garlic powder
1 tablespoon poultry
  seasoning

¼ cup finely chopped
  parsley
1 tablespoon grated
  Parmesan cheese
3 tablespoons sesame oil
½ cup grated Parmesan
  cheese

Rinse chicken breasts and pat dry with a paper towel. Combine paprika, onion powder, poultry seasoning, parsley and cheese in a small paper bag. Add chicken breasts one at a time and coat thoroughly with the mixture.

Heat a large nonstick pan over medium-high heat and add sesame oil. Swirl pan to coat evenly with oil. Add chicken breasts, being careful not to crowd pan, and sauté until chicken is evenly browned and cooked through.

Garnish generously with Parmesan cheese.

YIELD: 2 servings

Dill-Simmered Duck

1 duck (4 to 5 pounds)
2 cups strong beef stock
2 cloves garlic, minced
3 tablespoons dill weed

1 teaspoon paprika
Freshly ground black
   pepper, to taste

Trim off duck neck and discard. Remove and set aside giblets. Cut duck into serving size pieces, discarding any lumps of fat. Rinse duck pieces in cold running water and pat dry with a paper towel.

Place giblets and all duck pieces in a large frying pan on medium heat. Cook uncovered until browned on all sides, about 30 to 40 minutes. Remove duck pieces from pan and set aside. Pour off and discard drippings until about 1/4 cup remains in pan.

Add remaining ingredients to drippings and simmer for 5 minutes to combine flavors. Return duck to pan, reduce heat to low and simmer covered until meat is tender when pierced with fork, about 1 hour.

YIELD: 4 servings

FOURTEEN

Bread

Delicious salt-free breads are simple to make. The primary purpose salt serves in bread making is to retard the action of the yeast. Unsalted bread dough may rise excessively, so you should experiment. As you adapt other recipes to make them salt-free, be sure to cut down either on the yeast or the rising time. Be particularly careful about the final rise. If permitted to rise for too long, the bread may explode when the yeast is activated by the warmth of the oven!

Bagels

ॐ

1 package active dry yeast   *½ cup whole-wheat flour*
1½ cups warm water   *1 tablespoon bran*
4 cups unbleached flour   *6 quarts boiling water*

Dissolve yeast in ½ cup warm water. Cover, put in a warm place and let stand 15 minutes.

Mix flours and bran. Add yeast mixture and remaining 1 cup warm water to the flour-bran mixture to make a soft dough.

Knead for 5 minutes on floured board. Cover dough and let rise 15 minutes. Punch dough down, divide into 8 to 10 pieces. Roll each piece into a short, fat rope and join ends together to form circles of dough. Cover and let rise another 20 minutes.

Preheat oven to 350°F.

Drop bagels into boiling water; boil for one minute. Transfer to ungreased nonstick cookie sheet.

Bake for 30 minutes or until browned.

YIELD: 8 to 10 bagels

Variation: Onion Bagels

Sauté ¼ cup chopped onion in unsalted butter and sprinkle on bagels before baking.

French Bread

(Baguette [Long, Thin Loaf] and Pain de Campagne [Round Peasant Loaf])

Anyone who has ever been to France and eaten the bread can never forget the delicious crustiness of a real French baguette. The twofold secret of baking such good bread at home is to bake it on a rack lined with terra-cotta tiles and to spray it with water to create humidity as it bakes. These two simple procedures will be your way to a sensational loaf of French bread.

⅓ cup warm water	*4 cups bread flour*
1 package active dry	*(or 3 cups bread flour*
yeast (or 1 cake	*and 1 cup whole-wheat*
compressed fresh	*flour)*
yeast)	*1½ cups tepid water*

In an 8-ounce glass measuring cup, put ⅓ cup warm water. Be certain the water is not above 110°F (warm to the touch) for dry yeast or 95°F for cake yeast. Higher temperatures will kill the yeast. Stir the yeast into the water until smooth and set aside.

Place the flour in a large bowl. Make a well in the center and pour the 1½ cups tepid water into it. Add yeast-and-water mixture and begin scooping the flour into the liquid, mixing quickly with your fingers until the dough sticks together in a single mass.

Place the dough on a floured surface and knead. This is a soft dough with a lovely texture that is easy to handle. If dough becomes sticky, flour your hands and the work surface, and continue kneading. As you work the dough, it will become smooth and elastic, and will spring back when poked. At that point the dough is ready for its first rising. (Up to this stage, you may also make the dough in a food processor. Follow instructions for **Mazel Pizza** dough.)

Place dough in a buttered bowl. Turn to coat entire mass of dough with butter. Cover with a kitchen towel and set aside to rise. The rising time will depend on the warmth of the kitchen. Dough should double in size in about 2 hours.

Once dough has doubled, punch down, turn dough in bowl to grease it again and allow to rise again until doubled. The second rise should take a little less time. If, however, you wish to retard the rise, refrigerate dough. Simply remove from refrigerator whenever you're ready and let the dough double in size. After dough has risen a second time, punch down again and remove to a floured surface.

Baguettes

Flatten dough and with a large knife cut into three pieces, much longer than they are wide. To form the dough into a baguette, roll it with your hands from the center to the ends, your hands working in opposite directions. Make three long, skinny loaves. As they are formed, either place them on a floured cookie sheet or in a lightly floured French baguette-baking tin for the final rise. Cover with a kitchen towel and allow to rise for no more than $1/2$ hour. The final rise occurs rather quickly in salt-free bread.

Meanwhile, line oven rack with terra-cotta tiles. These are available in 6-inch squares from any ceramic tile store. Preheat the oven to 425°F and fill a spray bottle with tap water. Flour the tiles.

With a quick jerking motion, roll bread directly onto preheated tiles or place baguette tin on tiles. Spray baguettes lightly with water two or three times and close oven. After 10 minutes, spray again. Bake for 30 minutes or until bread is brown and sounds hollow when tapped on the bottom.

Pain de Campagne

To make a loaf of pain de campagne, do not cut in three when shaping loaves for the final rise. Simply roll the dough into a ball, place on floured cookie sheet to rise and cover with a towel. Bake directly on tiles and spray as for baguettes.

YIELD: 3 baguettes or 1 large round loaf

Bread Crumbs

To make bread crumbs, use day-old French bread—preferably your own. Cut into large cubes, place in a food processor or blender, and process or blend until reduced to tiny crumbs. You may add dried herbs to the bread crumbs (for example, parsley, oregano, basil or thyme). Store in an airtight container until ready to use.

Sage and Ginger Bread

This bread makes delicious toast topped with sweet butter. To save time, I make it in a food processor. If you prefer to knead by hand, the proportions are the same.

1 package active dry
* yeast (or 1 cake*
* compressed fresh yeast)*
⅓ cup warm water
1½ cups tepid water
1 teaspoon grated fresh
* ginger (more if you like*
* the zing)*
2 tablespoons fresh sage
* (or 1 tablespoon dried)*

2 tablespoons fresh
* oregano (or 1 table-*
* spoon dried)*
2 tablespoons light-
* colored sesame oil*
2 cups unbleached
* white or bread flour*
2 cups whole-wheat
* flour*

Dissolve the yeast in ⅓ cup water not above 110°F (warm to the touch) for dry yeast or 95°F for fresh. Place in a food processor or electric mixer equipped with a dough hook. Add 1½ cups tepid water, ginger, sage, oregano and oil. Process or beat for 30 seconds. Add the flours, 1 cup at a time, making sure each cup is thoroughly incorporated before adding the next cup. If the dough appears very moist, add more flour. Process or beat until the dough forms a ball.

Flour your hands and work surface, remove the dough from the processor or mixer, and knead for 1 minute or so—until you have a smooth, malleable mass.

Place in a greased bowl and allow to rise until doubled in bulk (approximately 2 hours). Punch down and allow to rise until doubled again (about 1 hour). Punch down again.

Remove from bowl to floured work surface and divide in two. Roll and shape into two loaves. Place in greased bread pans or make loaves round and free-form, peasant style. Cover with a towel and allow to rise for 1 hour, or until nearly doubled in size.

Bake in a preheated 350°F oven for about 45 minutes or until nearly doubled in size.

YIELD: 2 loaves

GROWING HERBS: *Herbs are fun to grow, and since most are used in relatively small amounts, it's practical to grow your own. All you need is a sunny windowsill. They can be preserved in rice vinegar for use in winter. Tarragon preserved in this way is especially delightful in hollandaise sauce. The vinegar flavor of the preserved herb is delicious.*

Rye Bread

Serve this flavorful bread with lots of sweet butter.

2 tablespoons unsalted
  butter
½ cup heavy cream
½ cup water
1 package active dry
  yeast (or 1 cake com-
  pressed fresh yeast)
1 cup warm water
3 cups unbleached white
  or bread flour
1¼ cups finely minced
  onion

3 tablespoons and 1 pinch
  caraway seeds
3 tablespoons chopped
  fresh dill (or 1½ tablespoons dried)
½ teaspoon ground
  cardamom
1½ cups rye flour
1 tablespoon cornmeal
1 tablespoon water

In a saucepan, melt butter. Add cream and ½ cup water to the same pan. Heat just until tepid; remove from heat.

Dissolve yeast in 1 cup warm water (not above 110°F if using dry yeast, 95°F if using fresh) and combine with cream-and-butter mixture. Place in a large mixing bowl and stir in the unbleached or bread flour. Stir in onion, 3 tablespoons caraway seeds, dill and cardamom. Add 1 cup rye flour and beat to combine.

Turn out onto a floured surface and knead until smooth and elastic (about 10 minutes). As the dough becomes more moist during kneading, add the extra ½ cup rye flour and work it into the dough.

Grease a large bowl with butter, place dough in

bowl and turn to coat entire mass of dough with but-ter. Cover with plastic wrap and let rise until doubled in bulk (1 to 2 hours, depending on the temperature of your kitchen).

When fully risen, punch down. Allow to rise again until doubled in bulk.

Again punch down and turn out onto a floured surface.

Press dough into a rectangle of about 9 x 6 inches. With a large knife dipped in flour, cut dough into two equal pieces. Begin working one piece of the dough into a ball, pinching it in at the bottom and pulling to round out the top. Repeat with other piece of dough.

Sprinkle cornmeal on a cookie sheet. Place both loaves on it and brush dough with 1 tablespoon water. Sprinkle a pinch of caraway seeds on loaf tops, cover with a kitchen towel and set aside to rise for about 35 to 45 minutes.

Preheat oven to 350°F.

Place loaves in oven and bake for 1 hour or until they are brown and sound hollow when rapped on the bottom. Set aside to cool.

YIELD: 2 loaves

FIFTEEN

Globe-Trotting and Table-Hopping

(Famous Chefs Spill the Beans)

In *The New Beverly Hills Diet*, I offered you the chance of a lifetime! It's the chance to be thin for life simply by taking charge of the food you eat. Let me remind you one more time: If you follow the rules of Conscious Combining as laid out in *The New Beverly Hills Diet*, not only will you become a Born-Again Skinny, you will embrace healthful and joyful eating habits that will keep you slim forever.

As I said in the beginning of this book, an important part of taking charge of the food you eat is coming to terms with the joy food brings into our lives. Too often, "diets" fail because they take the joy out of eating. An important part of this joy is the comfort we find in preparing familiar dishes—and the excitement we find in new dishes.

In this chapter, we'll look at how to adapt recipes to *The New Beverly Hills Diet*. To show you how easy it is, I'll share dishes from some of the glorious restaurants I've dined in while touring. You'll find two versions of each dish. The first recipe is the dish as prepared at the restaurant. The second recipe is a version adhering to the principles of Conscious Combining.

I promise you, when you realize how little the flavors and textures of a dish are affected by thoughtfully eliminating or replacing a few ingredients, you won't hesitate to begin making recipes from every cookbook on your shelves your own!

Recipe Rules

In adapting any recipe you must observe the essential principles of Conscious Combining. They're easy to remember and easy to follow:

- Proteins go with proteins; carbohydrates go with carbohydrates; fruit must be eaten alone.
- Carbohydrates are carbohydrates—whether starch, vegetable, salad, cereal or grain—and, for the most part, they should not be combined with proteins.
- Proteins are proteins—whether meat, fish, milk, yogurt, cheese, nut, seed or ice cream—and, for the most part, they should not be combined with carbohydrates.
- Fats such as butter, oil, mayonnaise, sour cream and heavy cream can be combined with either proteins or carbohydrates but not with fruit.

Skinny Recipe Tips

Select the recipes you alter with reasonable care. While nearly any recipe can be adapted to Conscious Combining, you'll get the best results with recipes that do not depend on critical ingredients that must be replaced for their distinctive character. For instance, don't expect your favorite fish dish to taste the same without the fruit salsa.

Many recipes can be adapted simply by eliminating the salt. To replace the flavor-enhancing quality of salt, add a sprinkling of rice vinegar to carbs, or add freshly ground pepper, a dash of grated fresh ginger or a pinch of minced fresh herbs to any serving. Salt-free prepared seasonings are becoming more and more popular—and widely available. One of my favorites is Mrs. Dash.

Salt, preservatives and other chemicals are pervasive in processed foods. When adapting a recipe or creating your own, avoid taking shortcuts with bottled sauces and flavorings unless they are sodium free. This will be boldly stated on the front label. Instead, use "whole" ingredients whenever possible.

For time-saving prepared ingredients, check out the products offered at health food stores and in the natural foods sections of supermarkets, but don't assume that "natural" means healthful or no-salt. You must be careful to thoroughly read ingredient lists on labels. Never assume any prepared food is no-salt unless it says so on the label!

Cape Cod Scallops Sauté au Citron

From The Blue Fox, San Francisco

2 pounds bay scallops	¹/₂ teaspoon Worcestershire
Flour	sauce
1 cup oil	Salt and pepper, to taste
¹/₄ pound (1 stick) butter	6 slices toast
2 large lemons	Lemon wedges, for garnish
2 teaspoons chopped	Chopped parsley, for
parsley	garnish

Rinse bay scallops and pat dry in a paper towel. Dredge in flour and shake vigorously to remove excess.

In a heavy sauté skillet, add enough cooking oil to fill to a ¹/₄-inch depth. Place skillet on medium-high heat. When oil is very hot, add the scallops. Let them brown very lightly for about 1 minute. Pour off all oil and add butter. Sauté scallops until butter is light brown.

Remove skillet from stove and add lemon juice and 2 teaspoons parsley. Add Worcestershire sauce, salt and pepper. Place on slices of toast. Garnish with lemon wedges and parsley.

YIELD: 6 servings

Scallops à la Conscious Combining

2 pounds bay scallops
8 tablespoons butter
½ cup minced shallot
4 cloves garlic, minced or
  pressed

4 tablespoons minced
  parsley

Rinse scallops and pat dry with paper towels. Remove any tough nibs that once attached scallops to their shells.

In a large sauté pan, heat butter until it foams. Add shallot and garlic, and sauté until very lightly browned. Add scallops, raise heat and sauté very quickly.

To ensure scallops cook evenly, jerk pan sharply every few seconds to keep scallops tossing and turning. Do not overcook—the entire cooking time should be no more than 3 minutes.

Arrange on a serving platter and top with parsley.

Note: Soft-shell crabs can be sautéed in the same manner. Simply increase the cooking time to 5 minutes on each side.

YIELD: 4 servings

Chicken Paillard with Rosemary Butter

From Mortimer's, New York City

Rosemary butter:

½ pound (2 sticks) unsalted
    butter
⅓ cup Dijon mustard

1 teaspoon coarsely
    chopped dried rosemary
1 teaspoon dried marjoram

Cream butter with mustard; add herbs. Wrap in foil and shape into a roll. Freeze.

YIELD: 4 servings

Chicken:

1 4- to 5-ounce chicken
    breast, skinned and
    boned
1 tablespoon butter, melted

Salt and pepper, to taste
Grilled tomato halves and
    watercress, for garnish

Place chicken breast, fillet side up, between two sheets of plastic wrap. Beat gently with a mallet until meat is evenly spread and about ⅛-inch thick. Brush with butter and seasonings.

Cook quickly over a very hot charcoal grill or in a very hot, well-oiled iron skillet.

Cut a ¼-inch slice or two of rosemary butter and serve with chicken. Garnish with grilled tomato halves and watercress.

YIELD: 1 serving

Chicken Paillard with Rosemary Butter à la Conscious Combining

Simply eliminate the salt in the original recipe. When making the rosemary butter, replace the Dijon mustard with dry mustard made into a paste with chicken broth or use the low-sodium variety of Dijon mustard available in health food stores.

YIELD: 1 serving

Terrine de Légumes
From *Le Cirque, New York City*

9 ounces artichoke bottoms
  (8 to 10, enough to make
  one layer in your pan)
6 ounces snow peas
6 ounces broccoli
6 ounces carrots, shredded
7 ounces knob celery,
  shredded

5 ounces red bell pepper,
  skinless
4 ounces green asparagus
  tips
Salt and pepper, to taste
8 sheets plain gelatin
4 ounces carrot juice
Vinaigrette sauce

Boil artichoke bottoms for 12 minutes. Steam remaining vegetables for 5 minutes. Add salt and pepper. Set vegetables aside to cool.

Presoak gelatin sheets in cold water, then mix with carrot juice. Heat for 10 seconds.

In a 4-pound mold pan, alternate layers of vegetables and gelatin. Refrigerate for 6 hours. Serve with a vinaigrette sauce.

YIELD: 20 slices

Terrine de Légumes à la Conscious Combining

The secret of a beautifully presented vegetable terrine is in the vegetables. Cut all the vegetables so they are of uniform size, both in width and length.

½ pound string beans, washed and ends snipped off
¾ pound carrots (as close in size and straight as possible)
6 artichokes
1 large cauliflower
2 tablespoons unsalted butter
2 tablespoons flour

½ cup heavy cream
2 egg yolks
1 teaspoon fresh tarragon (or ½ teaspoon dried)
¼ teaspoon cayenne pepper
Freshly ground or grated nutmeg, to taste
Freshly ground white pepper, to taste
Mayonnaise or **Beurre Blanc**

Fill a large pot with water and bring to a boil. Cook string beans for 5 minutes, or until crisp-tender. Refresh under cold water.

Scrape carrots and boil whole for 7 to 8 minutes, depending on width. Remove from boiling water and plunge into cold water. Slice into long, thin julienne strips.

Trim tops of artichokes. Cook trimmed artichokes in boiling water for 30 minutes. Drain, remove choke and trim leaves until you are left with just the bottoms. Trim bottoms as evenly as possible.

Wash cauliflower, cut into small florets and cook in

boiling water until tender when pierced with a fork. Drain thoroughly. Puree in a food processor or mill.

Melt butter in a small saucepan; add flour and whisk until foamy. Off the heat, add cream and, whisking constantly, return saucepan to stove and cook at a low boil until the mixture thickens. (This béchamel mixture will hold the terrine together.) When it has thickened, add cauliflower puree and stir until well blended. Beat in egg yolks. Season mixture with tarragon, cayenne, nutmeg and white pepper.

Butter a ½-quart loaf pan or terrine. Cut 1 green bean into tiny strips and small carrot rounds into flowers. Decorate bottom of terrine with these tiny flower carrots on long green stems made from string beans. Refrigerate terrine mold to harden butter and set flowers.

Remove terrine mold from refrigerator. Pour the first ½-inch layer of cauliflower mixture into terrine. Then add artichoke hearts set closely together, followed by another layer of cauliflower, a flat row of green beans, more cauliflower, the carrots placed side by side as tightly as possible, more cauliflower, green beans and, lastly, cauliflower.

Bake in a bain-marie (or casserole filled with boiling water to two-thirds of the way up the sides of the terrine) in a 350°F oven for 25 minutes or until a knife inserted in the center comes out clean. Cool and refrigerate until ready to serve. Serve from the terrine or invert onto a serving platter. Pass with a flavored mayonnaise or serve warm with beurre blanc.

YIELD: 6 to 8 servings

Oven-Roasted Eggplant Napoleon

From Kapalua Bay Hotel and Villas, Maui

I've included this delightful recipe from Anthony Edington, a talented chef at Maui's Kapalua Bay Hotel and Villas. This deliciously dish needs only a slight change. To make it work for Conscious Combining and *you*, just replace the balsamic vinegar with rice vinegar . . . then enjoy!

Tomato coulis:

8 large plum tomatoes
3 tablespoons extra-virgin olive oil
1 Maui onion (or any sweet onion such as Vidalia)
8 cloves garlic
1 teaspoon chopped fresh thyme

1 teaspoon chopped fresh oregano
1 tablespoon balsamic vinegar
Freshly ground black pepper, to taste

Preheat oven to 350°F.

Remove stem ends of tomatoes and cut tomatoes in half. Spread oil on a small sheet pan and place cut tomato on top. Cut onion into ½-inch rings and place on sheet pan with tomatoes. Remove root stem from garlic and place garlic on the sheet pan. Sprinkle all with thyme and oregano.

Bake for 15 minutes or until onion just starts to

blacken (past brown so vegetables start to caramelize). Puree in blender until smooth.

Add balsamic vinegar and pepper.

Roasted red peppers:
2 red bell peppers

Place peppers on a sheet pan under a hot broiler and broil until skin is blistered and blackened. Rotate pepper to roast evenly on all sides.

Remove peppers from oven, place in a bowl and cover with plastic wrap. Allow to cool, then remove skin, slice open, and remove seeds and membranes. Slice into strips and reserve for garnish.

Eggplant:

2 large eggplants	*4 tablespoons extra-virgin*
2 tablespoons finely	*olive oil*
chopped garlic	*1 green zucchini*
4 tablespoons chopped	*1 yellow zucchini*
fresh basil	*4 sprigs fresh basil*

Preheat oven to 325°F.

Slice eggplants into ¹/₂-inch rounds. Place on a nonstick sheet pan. In a small bowl combine garlic, basil and oil; mix well. Evenly distribute mixture on each piece of eggplant.

Slice green and yellow zucchini into ¹/₄-inch rounds. Place green zucchini on eggplant in a single layer to cover half of the eggplant. Cover remaining half with yellow zucchini in single layer.

Bake in oven for 15 to 20 minutes until eggplant is soft.

Place 3 eggplant rounds one on top of the other, alternating colors of zucchini. Decorate with roasted bell pepper strips and basil sprigs.

Place one-quarter of tomato coulis and one layered round on each of four plates.

YIELD: 4 servings

Chutneys Cauliflower with Potatoes

I was blessed to find myself living next door to one of Seattle's hottest restaurants—and one particularly suited to Conscious Combining. Chutneys serves Indian cuisine like none I have ever tasted. Fresh, delicious and healthful, it was my lunchtime indulgence. Their food made my day—almost every day! This delightfully simple and flavorful recipe was adapted without salt by Chutneys especially for Conscious Combining.

2 tablespoons sesame oil	½ teaspoon black pepper
½ teaspoon cumin seed	2 medium-size potatoes,
1 yellow onion, sliced	steamed and quartered
1 green chile, split	1 pound cauliflower florets,
1 teaspoon minced fresh	blanched
ginger	Garam masala
½ teaspoon cayenne	Cilantro sprigs
powder	1 tomato, diced

In a heavy-bottomed sauté pan, heat oil until hot, add cumin seed. When cumin seed is browned, add onion and chile. Cook until onion is translucent. Add ginger, cayenne powder and black pepper, and stir in potato. Cook potatoes for 2 to 3 minutes, then add cauliflower florets and heat through. Sprinkle with garam masala, and garnish with cilantro sprigs and diced tomato.

YIELD: 2 servings

Reading a Restaurant Menu Through the Eyes of a Born-Again Skinny

Trying to "play it straight" in a restaurant might seem complicated at first, but after you've done it once, you won't have to think twice!

To make your restaurant forays easier, I've included this menu as an example of how to make their food work for you. All you have to do is read the menu carefully and ask your waitperson a few questions if the menu isn't clear about ingredients. Don't try to second-guess or assume. If you aren't sure, ask. Then it's just a matter of mix and match, pick and choose, or leaving out a few foods. You can almost always adapt the toughest menus to your new Skinny ways.

P denotes a protein dish.

C denotes a carbohydrate dish.

X denotes an entity unto itself: an inherent mis-combination . . . it is what it is and there is no getting away from it. The protein and carbohydrates are joined at the hip and cannot be separated.

To avoid a miscombination, you should avoid the portion of a dish that I've crossed out. It's best to ask the waitperson to leave the offending food *off* the plate. Don't tempt fat or temptation—I don't! At the very least, you can give it to someone else or take it home and include it in your next carbohydrate meal. Note that I said *carbohydrate meal*—that's because you should only do this with a dish that you wish to turn into an all-protein dish. *Never* do this with a dish you want to convert to an all-carbohydrate meal. The protein portion of the dish will have permeated the very soul of the carbohydrates and rendered them a miscombination.

If you are following the 80/20 protein rule, then go ahead and enjoy a bit of the carbohydrate, but don't get carried away—or you soon will be carried "a-weigh" to your former weight.

Last but certainly not least: One of my favorite dishes (and probably one of yours) is pizza. Unfortunately, by its very nature, this luscious mix of carbs and proteins is a glaring miscombination. So what to do? Give up pizza? NEVER!

Don't think ordering a vegetarian pizza gives you an easy way out or is a "better" choice . . . it only adds insult to injury. Unless this meatless dish is also *cheeseless*, you'll trap the crust and the whole load of vegetables. And don't try to pick the cheese out thinking you'll be able to remove every gooey bit. IMPOSSIBLE!

The best answer is to eat a *protein* pizza (unless, of course, a veggie pizza is your fave rave) so all that gets trapped is the crust. Eating the cheese, the topping and the back—or say one-fifth of—the crust keeps it within the confines of the 80/20 rule. If you eat only the cheese and the topping, you can make the pizza an all-protein dish.

---- STARTERS ----

Sausage and Roasted Peppers—P
Sweet and spicy Italian sausage, ~~roasted peppers and caramelized onions, tossed in a marinara sauce over linguine.~~

Fried Calamari—P
Tossed in a spicy batter, fried in canola oil, served with chilled cocktail sauce and garlic mayonnaise.

Bagna Calda—P
Whole roasted garlic served with Roma tomatoes, fresh basil, olive oil and warm pizza bread.

Garlic Shrimp—P
Sautéed in a scampi sauce, and ~~served over black-and-white linguine.~~

Risotto*—C
Changes daily, please ask your server.

Antipasto—C
~~Fresh mozarella,~~ sliced Roma tomatoes and grilled eggplant, topped with fresh basil and extra-virgin olive oil.

Mushroom Ravioli—P
Served on fried spaghettini, topped with wild mushrooms in a light marsala cream sauce.

Shrimp Cocktail—P
Black tiger prawns poached in court bouillon, served with a spicy cocktail sauce.

Bruschetta—C
Fresh Roma tomatoes, basil, garlic and olive oil, served on toasted filone bread.

---

* With vegetables only. If it is protein, . . . pass.

SALADS

Caesar—C

Crisp romaine, seasoned croutons and ~~Parmesan cheese~~, all tossed in our Caesar dressing.

Garden—C

Seasonal vegetables, croutons and green onion on romaine, honey mustard or balsamic vinaigrette dressing served on the side.

Misto—C

Organic baby greens with julienne zucchini and carrots, ~~toasted walnuts and pine nuts,~~ tossed in balsamic vinaigrette.

Greens and Gorgonzola—C

Organic baby greens, ~~gorgonzola cheese~~, Roma tomatoes ~~and toasted walnuts~~, tossed in balsamic vinaigrette.

PIZZA

All pizzas are made with a blend of mozzarella and fontina cheeses.

Lox—P
Cured salmon, ~~red onion~~ and dilled cream cheese (served at room temperature).

Chicken Cilantro—P
Spicy chicken, cilantro, pesto, pico de gallo and sour cream.

Mediterranean
Pesto, artichoke hearts and sun-dried tomatoes.

Mushroom
Roasted garlic, oregano, and sautéed domestic and wild mushrooms.

Primavera Calzone
Artichoke hearts, zucchini, carrots and mushrooms, served with marinara.

Marciano
Sun-dried tomatoes, roasted garlic and fresh herbs.

Misto—P
Blackforest ham, ~~zucchini~~, goat cheese and roasted garlic.

Barbequed Chicken—P
Spicy chicken in barbecue sauce with ~~red onions~~ and cilantro.

Mexican Sausage—P
Chicken sausage, ~~red onion~~, smoked gouda cheese and cilantro.

Garden
Grilled radicchio, fresh spinach, roasted garlic and goat cheese.

Margherita
Roma tomatoes and fresh basil (with your choice of olive oil or tomato sauce base).

Cheese—P
With tomato sauce.

VEGETARIAN PASTAS

Mediterranean Pasta—C
Artichoke hearts, sun-dried tomatoes, mushrooms and pesto, tossed with fettuccine.

Vegetarian Lasagna
Layers of seasonal vegetables, herbed ricotta cheese and marinara between spinach-and-egg pasta, with garlic cream and fresh tomatoes.

Pasta Primavera—C
Seasonal vegetables, fresh basil, black olives and tomatoes, in olive oil and garlic over spinach linguine.

Fettuccine Alfredo
Fettuccine in a cream and Parmesan cheese sauce.

Red Bell Pepper Ravioli
With spicy chicken, red onion, bell peppers and cilantro pesto.

Penne Arrabiata—C
Penne with Roma tomatoes and fresh basil, in a spicy marinara sauce.

Lemon-Pepper Fettuccine—C
Sun-dried tomatoes and broccoli, tossed in olive oil and garlic, topped with goat cheese.

Garden Farfalle—C
Grilled radicchio, fresh spinach and red onion, tossed in olive oil and garlic, topped with fresh basil and goat cheese.

Cheese and Spinach Cannelloni—C
Stuffed with ricotta cheese and fresh spinach, topped with pesto, marinara and garlic cream sauces.

Wild Mushroom Ravioli—C
Tossed in a sun-dried tomato-basil cream sauce.

Farfalle Morbidella—C
Farfalle with sautéed eggplant, tossed in a checca sauce and topped with fresh morbidella cheese.

Basil Spaghettini Checca—C
Olive oil and garlic, Roma tomatoes and basil.
Add goat cheese, chicken or shrimp.

PASTA SPECIALTIES

Cajun Chicken—P
Spicy chicken in our garlic cream,
~~with red bell pepper fettuccine,~~
~~topped with green onions.~~

Stuffed Chicken Breast—P
Stuffed with herbed ricotta and pine
nuts, ~~on a bed of linguine with~~
~~pesto.~~

Italian Sausage and Roasted Peppers—P
Sweet and spicy sausage, ~~roasted~~
~~peppers, caramelized onions~~ and
Parmesan cheese, ~~on a bed of~~
~~linguine.~~

Pasta Puttanesca
Black olive, capers, tomatoes and
anchovies, in a red wine and butter
sauce on lemon-pepper fettuccine.

Penne Amatriciana
Pancetta, red onion, garlic and red
pepper flakes, in a red wine and
herb-butter sauce.

Chicken Marsala—P
Two chicken breasts seared, with
~~sautéed mushrooms~~ and marsala
wine sauce, ~~on a bed of linguine.~~

Penne with Mexican Sausage—P
Chicken sausage, ~~red onion,~~
~~tomatoes~~ with olive oil and garlic,
topped with smoked gouda and
cilantro.

Santa Fe Ravioli
Chicken ravioli, in our garlic cream
sauce, tossed with pico de gallo
salsa.

Shrimp, Pesto and Goat Cheese—P
~~Served on a bed of linguine~~ with
toasted pine nuts.

Misto Chicken—P
Grilled breasts with ~~red onion,~~
~~tomatoes~~ and basil, in a marinara
and red wine sauce, ~~on tomato~~
~~fettuccine.~~

Chicken Cilantro Ravioli
Tossed in a cilantro cream sauce,
topped with Roma tomatoes and
green onions.

Garlic Shrimp—P
Sautéed in herb butter, garlic
and brandy, served over ~~black-~~
~~and-white spaghetti.~~

Lobster Ravioli
Served with your choice of a checca
sauce or caper-and-cream sauce.

New York Steak—P
Grilled, and topped with ~~mushroom~~
~~caps, caramelized onions~~ and herb
butter, ~~on lemon-pepper fettuccine.~~

Smoked Salmon Ravioli

Index

249

THE *New* BEVERLY HILLS DIET Skinny Shop

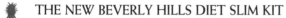

Featuring a selection of exciting products and services
for the new Slim you, including:

THE NEW BEVERLY HILLS DIET SLIM KIT
Let Judy personally guide you through each of the 35 days with this
four audio-cassette program.

CLUBSLIM MEMBERSHIP
Be a part of Judy's personal support network.

THE NEW BEVERLY HILLS DIET SKINNY SURVIVAL KIT
The highest quality unsulfured dried fruits and unrefined oils.
All you'll need for the 35 days of the diet (plus one for the road).
Individual items also available.

THE BORN-AGAIN SKINNY SCALE
The very same scale that Judy uses each day. So small it even fits in
a suitcase!

THE NEW BEVERLY HILLS DIET SKINNY SUPPLEMENTS
Healthful additions to your new Slim eating program.

SKINNY INSURANCE
Personal and private support is just a phone call away.

THE BEVERLY HILLS DIET
A special edition of the original 1981 blockbuster!

For more information about these and other *New Beverly Hills Diet*
products, or to place your order:

Call: (310) 573-4263
Write: Judy Mazel, 17250 Sunset Blvd., #301, Pacific Palisades, CA 90272
Internet: www.cyberskinny.com

Be sure to inquire about special savings on Skinny Packages!

Discover the Slim New You!

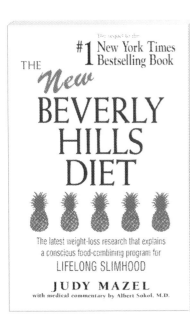

The New Beverly Hills Diet

Now you can enjoy your favorite foods—from steak and pasta to champagne and chocolate—and still lose weight easily. Judy Mazel shows you how! Supported by medical credentials, the secret to this program is Conscious Combining, the technique that teaches you how and when to mix different food groups for optimum weight control. You'll learn, once and for all, how to indulge in your favorite food fantasies without packing on the pounds. **#4258—$12.95**

The New Beverly Hills Diet
Little Skinny Companion

Need a little extra help? In addition to containing affirmations to help you start each day off right, this book also provides you with plenty of helpful reminders to keep you on track! You'll find the Golden Rules of the program, a 35-day diet list, corrective counterparts to remedy miscombined meals, food group classifications and a daily diary for charting your daily progress. Just the friend you need on your journey to lifelong slimhood! **#4762—$4.95**

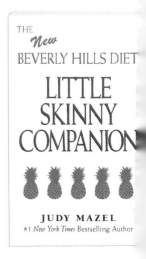

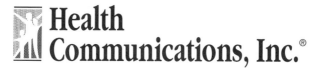
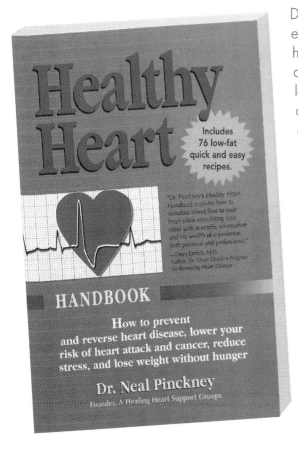

Books to Nurture Your Body & Soul!

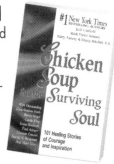
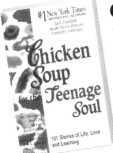
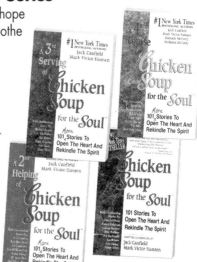